From The Kitchen of New Hope Church

Dr. Betty Glover Perry

Order this book online at www.trafford.com
or email orders@trafford.com

Most Trafford titles are also available at major online book retailers.

Printed in the United States of America.

ISBN: 978-1-4269-6168-7 (sc)
ISBN: 978-1-4269-6169-4 (e)

Trafford rev. 03/16/2011

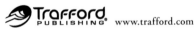 www.trafford.com

North America & International
toll-free: 1 888 232 4444 (USA & Canada)
phone: 250 383 6864 ♦ fax: 812 355 4082

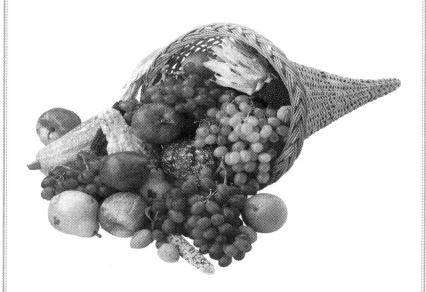

A plant-based diet will not make one weak. Horsepower has been used to describe the speed of locomotives. The horse is a very strong and useful animal, and only eats vegetation.

From the kitchen of New Hope Church

W elcome to the world of healthfully delicious eating for the new vegetarian. Professional dietetic organizations have stated that a vegetarian diet can provide all of the nutrients needed for abundant health. (The American Dietetic Association Foundation) A nutritious diet is one that contains daily servings from the Basic Four Food Group:

Meat or Protein 2		2 oz. servings
Milk 2		1 cup servings
Fruit and Vegetables 4		½ c servings
Bread and Cereal 4		servings

All vegetation consists of partial proteins; thus two vegetables from different sources will equal a complete protein. A combination of beans and bread are a complete protein source. Beans, milk, cheese, legume and nuts are the protein sources used in this book.

The heart and dietetic association's recommends that animal fats and hard fats be eliminated and the use of vegetables oils, with fewer servings of cream, salt and eggs are better choices for healthful living.

Over 50% of the recipes in this book use commercial meat analogs (textured vegetable protein or TVP). The analogs are designed to taste similar to the product it replaces. These products are readily available in the local chain grocery supermarkets and health food stores.

The TVP'S used in these recipes are supplied by Kellogg's Natural and Frozen Food Division: Morningstar Farms, Loma Linda, Natural Touch, Worthington and Eggo. All recipes that used TVP's are acknowledged with a *.

The Church family wished you and your loved ones **Bon Appétit** as you enjoy these new flavors, textures and taste.

Our Mission
09/09/2010

One can choose their own health-wise lifestyle by changing habits.

Cutting the fat by cutting back on meat reduces the risk of heart disease and automatically reduces the fat consumed by eating more vegetarian meals. By making the cut in meat eating and replacing it slowly and gradually with foods which are healthier, one can live better, healthier, wiser, happier and longer. (American Heart Association)

Getting the most out of one's diet by the right choices of foods is the first step to a complimentary healthy lifestyle. Beginning in the kitchen and getting back to basics. Include foods that consist of nuts, grains, fruits and vegetables are the cutting edge to a healthy by choice lifestyle.

Consider this, healthy foods that are an alternative to the most popular western diet which consists basically of meats, high in protein, saturated fats, animal fats, high in cholesterol. A defense against heavy weight, heart disease, strokes, high blood pressure, diabetes, kidney failure, cancer and much more starts in the kitchen. (*The American Dietetic Association*)

Try using spicy seasons such as lemon, lime, garlic, jalapeno with other green and red peppers, onions, salsa to add a zing or zestful flavor and sea salt.

Make the salad connection by adding raw foods as a daily part of the diet. The use of olive oil and vegetable oils are a better choice than the saturated fats like lard. Butter, margarine and vegetable oils should be used in moderation.

The purpose of this book is to help the beginning vegetarian get started by making a switch from animal flesh to a non-flesh plant based diet. Alternative foods that are prepared in a tasty, not bland way, prepared in a nourishing way for a healthier and better YOU.

An old saying, but true," what goes around, comes around". (Waylon Jennings, RCA Victor, 1979) Yes even in health care we reap the harvest of what we sow, genetic, heredity, our choices of lifestyle or a combination of all three may equal poor health.

Cookbook Committee

Editor

Dr. Betty Glover Perry

Committee Chairpersons

Ms. Irene Williams...................Publicity and Distribution

Ms. Rudene Morton............................Selection and Testing

Ms. Mary Alford.............Selection and Testing

Ms. Naomi Thompson..............Composition

Ms. Martha Bethea.............Secretarial Consultant

Ms. Pelicia Bethea..........Secretarial Consultant

The Cookbook Committee extends its appreciation for all of the efforts to get this publication out in a timely manner. Each recipe submitted may not have originated with the donor; however our main interest is better nutritional health to the community.

This is a dual project of the Community Service ministry to raise funds and promote healthier eating in this rural town where the associated diseases of poor dietary habits are rampant. The recipes in this book are basically lacto-ova vegetarian (does not contain animal flesh, but may contain dairy products and eggs.)

We acknowledge all who assisted us with proofreading, typing and copying. This project was a team effort of the members of New Hope Church. To God we give all the praise, honor and glory, because we have a

New Hope!

A regular diet of fast foods, processed, greasy, salty and sugary foods is the fastest way to a chronic disease state in every age group."Unhealthy eating increases risks for chronic disease."(Youfa Wang, 2010)

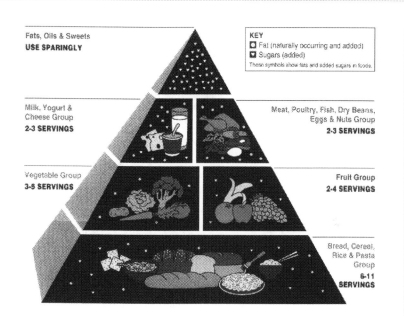

"The study shows that children with unfavorable overall school performance were more likely to eat sweets and fried foods, and were less likely to eat foods rich in protein, vitamins, and minerals." (Ming-Ling Fu, 2007) This is more reason to teach positive nutrition at home, and encourage it when away.

It is 2010, and there are more than enough scientific, medical and spiritual evidences to support a plant –based diet. Our Creator placed all the nutrients in plants, there is no reason to worry. Additionally, there are more familiar sources of protein such as nuts and beans. Complete proteins in whole grains, broccoli and potatoes. If you are just beginning you have plenty of options to get started and replace the meat. (Message, 2010)

About the author:

Dr. Betty Glover Perry, an anesthetist for 35 years, presently semi-retired and back in school, again. During the career noting the treatment of high blood pressure, multiple cardiovascular diseases and diabetes affect people of every walk in life. One common factor present in 99% of patients was a high meat and fatty diet.

Being a wife and mother, the goal was to prepare healthy tasty foods for family as well as raise the level of awareness of every person.

The cookbook idea is an endeavor to share with extended family and friends as well as the general public. Knowledge of one's eating habits contributes to the overall health. Our Creator has given us the gifts needed; we only need to avail ourselves of them. There are eight steps in the plan for overall better life. (E.G. White, 1942)

Nutritious food

Exercise

Water

Sunlight

Temperate

Sunlight

Air

Trust in Divine Power

Vegetarian diet: How to get the best nutrition

A well-planned vegetarian diet is a healthy way to meet your nutritional needs. Find out what you need to know about a plant-based diet.

You may follow a vegetarian diet for cultural, religious or ethical reasons. Or you may eat a vegetarian diet to stay healthy and prevent health problems, such as cardiovascular disease. Whatever your reasons for choosing a vegetarian diet, this guide will help you make smart choices to ensure that you meet your daily nutritional needs.

Indeed, a well-planned vegetarian diet can meet the needs of people of all ages, including children, teenagers, and pregnant or breast-feeding women. The key is to be aware of your nutritional needs so that you plan a diet that meets them. If you aren't sure how to create a vegetarian diet that's right for you, talk with your doctor and a registered dietitian.

Types of vegetarian diets

When people think about a vegetarian diet, they typically think about a diet that doesn't include meat, poultry or fish. But vegetarian diets can be further categorized into three types:

- **Vegan diets** exclude meat, poultry, fish, eggs and dairy products — and foods that contain these products.
- **Lacto-vegetarian diets** exclude meat, fish, poultry and eggs, as well as foods that contain them. Dairy products, such as milk, cheese, yogurt and butter, are allowed in a lacto-vegetarian diet.
- **Lacto-ova vegetarian diets** exclude meat, fish and poultry, but allow eggs and dairy products.

Some people follow a semi vegetarian diet — also called a flexi-tarian diet — which is primarily a plant-based diet but includes meat, dairy, eggs, poultry and fish on occasion or in small quantities.

Vegetarian diet pyramid

A healthy diet takes planning, and a food pyramid can be a helpful tool. The vegetarian pyramid outlines food groups and food choices that, if eaten in the right quantities, form the foundation of a healthy vegetarian diet. (Mayo Foundation, June 10, 2010)

References:

American Dietetic Association.
   http://www.eatright.org/ extracted, 09/2010

American Heart Association
   http://www.heart.org/HEARTORG/, 09/2010

Justin Timberlake, 2007) "What Goes Around Comes Around"

Kellogg's Natural and Frozen Food Division: *Morningstar Farms,*
   Loma Linda, 2010, Natural Touch, Worthington and Eggo.
   Battle Creek, Mi.

Mayo Foundation   June 10, 2010© 1998-2010   Medical
   Education and Research (MFMER).

Message Magazine, 2010   *Eat Complete without Meat, pg.18*
   Review and Herald Publishing
   Hagerstown, MD.

Ming-Ling Fu, 2007   *Dietary Intake Patterns of Low-Income*
   Urban African-American Adolescents
   Volume 110, Issue 9, Pages 1340-1345, September 2010

Youfa Wang, 2007   *The obesity epidemic in the United*
   States—gender, age, socioeconomic, racial/ethnic, and
   geographic characteristics:
   Johns Hopkins Bloomberg School of Public Health) 29: 6–28.

White, E.G.   1942   *Ministry of Healing*
   Review and Herald

TABLE OF CONTENTS

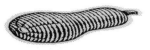

Bread

The aroma of fresh bread has become a reminder of generations gone by.

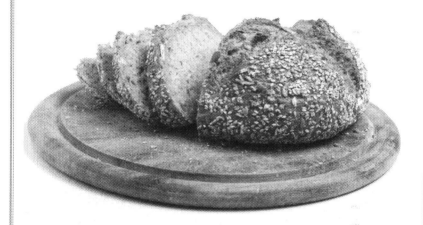

With current technology, bread making is not a lost art.

Here's a list of suggested toppers to make your bread extra special:

Herb Butter

Fruit Spreads

Herbal Spiced Oils

Dipping Sauce

Enjoy !!

Breakfast Brunch

Chili Cheddar Omelet

4 eggs	1T water
¼ t seasoned salt	1 c. chili
¼ c cheese, grated	
½ c avocado, sliced	

In small bowl beat eggs, water and seasoned salt together. Pour mixture into well buttered skillet.

Cook omelet over medium heat, letting liquid egg run to edges when eggs are set; slide omelet onto serving plate. Place chili, grated cheese and avocado slices on half of omelet and fold over the other half.

Serves: 2

Pumpkin Bread

4c flour	3 c sugar
2 t baking soda	1 ½ t salt
1 t baking powder	½ t cloves
1 t cinnamon/nutmeg	1 can pumpkin
¼ t ginger	1 c oil
4 eggs	2/3c water

Preheat oven to 350 degrees. Prepare 2 9x5x3 inch loaf pans.

Mix dry ingredients well then add moist ingredients and stir well. Do not over mix. Divide batter between the 2 prepared pans, bake at 350 degrees for 1 hour and 15 minutes.

Remove loaves from pan after 15 minutes.

Serves: 12   Ethel Bell

Puffy French toast

4 slices bread	½ c. milk
1 egg	¾ c biscuit mix
2 t. sugar	½ t. cinnamon
½ c. butter	

Melt butter in skillet on medium heat. With electric mixer, combine milk, egg, biscuit mix, sugar and cinnamon.

Cut each slice of bread in half diagonally. Dip bread in batter; coating completely. Fry 4 pieces at a time until golden brown and puffy.(about 3 minutes on each side).

Sprinkle with confectioner's sugar and cinnamon. Serve with warm syrup.

Serves: 2   Monique Perry Nervis

Blueberry Coffee Cake

2 c cake flour	1 c. sugar
1 t baking powder	2 eggs
1 t baking soda	1 t. vanilla
2 sticks butter	1.c. sour cream
1 can blueberry pie filling	

Preheat oven 375 degrees; prepare a 13x9x2 inch baking pan. Mix dry ingredients, then combine all ingredients except berries, blending well. Spoon half of batter in pan then pour blueberry pie filling, then top with remainder of batter. Bake for 40 minutes.

Breakfasts

Scrambled Tofu

¼ t. Spike seasoning

Heats until flavors are blended.

Breakfast Suggestions:

Scrambled tofu

Morningstar Farms "Links or strips"

Yellow grits

Toast

Serves: 4   Ethel Bell

Perry Breakfast

3 slices whole wheat bread, toasted

¼ c. peanut butter

2 c. apple sauce or apple butter

Margarine

Serve toast with margarine and/or peanut butter. Spoon heated applesauce over toast. Any fruit sauce will do. Serve with a glass of milk

Serves: 2   Betty Perry

Oatmeal Waffles

4 c. quick oats	3 c. hot water
½ c. powdered milk	¼ c. oil
1 t. salt	sesame seeds

Mix all ingredients thoroughly. Heat waffle iron and spray well with cooking spray. Place a large spoonful of batter on the waffle iron and closed the lid. Bake until brown, 5-7 minutes.

Serves: 4   Mary Brown

Southern Johnny cakes

2 c. corn meal   1 t. sea salt

3 T. margarine   2 T. Brown sugar

½ c. milk   2. C boiling water

Combine and drop by spoonfuls onto a greased griddle and flatten to ½ inch thick. Turn over when brown around edges. Serve with applesauce or syrup.

Serves: 2   Joann Barnes

Pancakes-Sausage

Pancake mix for 6   3 eggs

½ c. buttermilk   ½ c. olive oil

6 Morningstar Farms Breakfast Patties

Mix pancake batter with the eggs and buttermilk. Crumble the breakfast patties into the batter along with ½ of the oil. Drop by spoonfuls onto a hot griddle or fry pan, flipping once. Serve with syrup, honey or applesauce.

Serves: 3   Martha Bethea

Breakfast Brunch
*Wham Cheese Muffin

6 slices *Wham   6 slices cheese

Vegetable Spray   6 eggs

Can mushrooms   green onions, chopped

Salt and pepper

Spray muffin pan well. Arrange a slice of Wham into each cup of the muffin pan, topped by a slice of cheese. In a skillet sauté' onions and mushrooms then spoon this mixture into each of the cups and sprinkle with salt and pepper. Bake for 10 minutes at 350 degree.

Serves: 6   Joann Barnes

Breakfast Sandwich

4 hard boiled chopped eggs
4 Morningstar Breakfast Strips, browned and chopped
¼ c. mayo
1 c. Swiss cheese, grated
1 t. tarragon
1 ¼ t. Mustard
8 slices bread

Mix together all ingredients except bread. Spread the mixture evenly between 8 slices of bread, forming 4 sandwiches. Spread melted butter on outside surfaces of top and bottom of sandwiches. Brown on both sides in heavy skillet; then cut in half to serve.

Serves: 4   Mary Smith

Potato Croquettes

3 Potatoes, mashed   parsley diced
2Beaten eggs   salt & pepper to taste
Diced red peppers   cheese cut in inch strips

On well floured board, take a handful of the potato mixture and place on the board. Pat the potato ball until it is the size of a biscuit. Place the cheese   and *bacon-bits if desired in the center then start rolling up the potato into a roll.

Dip the roll in the beaten egg and then into the flour on all sides. Place the finished rolls into a hot fry pan with vegetable oil and fry on both sides until brown.

Serves: 3   Betty Perry

Salt Facts

Creative use of herbs and spices help eliminate added salt in recipes. USFDA recommends 2400 mg per day.
Tips for reducing salt intake:
Don't use herb salts like garlic salt or onion salt.
Don't salt during cooking: only at the end.
Don't salt cooking water.

Salads

Tricolored slaw

1 small head of red or green cabbage

(Or half of each)

2 lg. carrots, shredded

2 med. Apples, chopped

4 green onions, thinly slice, diagonal

1 c yogurt   ¼ c mayo

3 T. white wine vinegar

1 T sugar   ½ t. tarragon

Seasonings to taste

In large bowl combine the vegetables and refrigerate. In food processor combine remaining ingredients and blend well, pour over the vegetables and toss.

Serves: 6   Patricia Davis

Oriental Vegetable Salad

¼ c. cauliflower buds

¼ c. bean sprouts

Water chestnuts, thinly sliced

¼ c. cabbage, shredded

¼ c. mushrooms, fresh, sliced

¼ c. green onion, chopped

Italian dressing

Toss vegetables, add dressing and toss again.

Patricia Davis

Carrot Salad

1 can crushed pineapple

1 ½ c. carrots, shredded

¾ c flaked coconut

1 t. sugar

2 T. mayo

Combine all ingredients and mix well.

Serves: 4-6   Mary Smith

Orange Mallow Ambrosia

1 pkg. orange gelatin

¾ c. boiling water

2 c. ice cubes

1 c. whipped topping

1 can mandarin orange sections

c. miniature marshmallows

1 15oz. can crushed pineapple

Dissolve gelatin in boiling water. Add cubes and stir constantly until it starts to thicken. Add whipped topping, blending until smooth. Stir in oranges, marshmallows and pineapple and pour into mold or serving bowl. Chill until set.

Yield: 4 cups   Ethel Bell

Hot Cabbage Slaw

4 c cabbage, shredded

1 can green beans

¼ c sugars

1 t. minced onion

1 t. salt

½ c. vinegar

In saucepan, heat all ingredients to boiling, reduce heat, simmer, uncovered for 5 minutes more.

Ethel Bell

Green and Gold Salad

1 pkg.(10 oz.) green peas, frozen

½1 ½ t. Prepared mustard

c. cheese, shredded

2T. onion, chopped

2 T. mayo

1 ½ t. Prepared mustard

Seasonings

Crisp salad greens

Rinse green peas briefly in running cold water. Mix all ingredients except salad greens. Serve the salad on greens.

Easy Fruit Salad

1 c, seedless grapes

1 can mandarin oranges, drain

1 can pineapple chunks, drained

1 red apple, sliced

Yogurt dressing

Combine fruits and serve on salad greens with yogurt dressing.

Yogurt Dressing

2/3 c plain yogurt

1 T. honey

1 T. lemon juice

Mix all ingredients together.

Broccoli and Mushroom Salad

bunches fresh broccoli

1 lb. fresh mushrooms, sliced

1 bottle zesty Italian dressing

Cut broccoli into flowerets add mushrooms and dressing, cover and chill several hours.

24 Hour Salad

1 can pitted sweet cherries, drained

cans mandarin oranges

1 c miniature marshmallows

Old Fashion Fruit Dressing

Combine all ingredients, cover and chill for 12-24 hours.

Fruit Dressing:

2eggs, beaten	1 T. butter
2. T sugar	2 t lemon juice
2. T sugar	Dash of salt
2 c whipped topping	2 T fruit juice

Combine all ingredients except whipped topping in a saucepan, heat just to boiling. Remove from heat and cool. In a chilled bowl, fold in all ingredients.

Cucumber Salad

cucumbers, peeled and thinly sliced

¼ t. salt	2 T. vinegar
t. Lemon juice	½ t.dry mustard
T mayo or sour cream	
t. minced parsley	
3 t. green onion, chopped	

Place peeled cucumbers over the bottom of a colander and let drain for 30 minutes to remove excess liquid then chill. Mix remainder ingredients and toss into the cucumbers.

Spinach Corn Bread

1 onion, chopped
4 eggs
1 stick of butter
boxes Martha White cornbread mix
1 c. cottage cheese
dash salt
½ box frozen, chopped spinach

Mix together and bake in greased pan at 350 degrees until browned.

Bobbie Drummond

BREADS
Crackling Corn Bread

1 c. corn meal, self rising
½ c. oil
green onions chopped
3 eggs
1c butter milk
6 *Morningstar Farms breakfast strips

Chop breakfast strips and sauté in oil. Combine all ingredients and mix well. Pour into oiled baking pan. Bake at 350 for 35 minutes.
Serves: 8   Betty Perry

For variations a can or corn and crushed red peppers can be added to the batter. Also delicious when broccoli and cheese added to batter

Cottage Cheese Bread

2 eggs, beaten
c sugar   ¾ c milk
1 t vanilla   2 ¾ c flour
½ t baking powder   ½ c raisins
½ c nuts, chopped

Mix all together. Pour into an oiled pan and bake at 350 degrees for 60 Minutes.
                    Janet Taylor

GINGER MUFFINS

1 c butter   1 c sugar
1 c molasses   3 eggs
1 c buttermilk   13/4 t soda
2t ginger   2 t cinnamon
1 t nutmeg   ½ t salt
1 c flour   Cream butter and sugar. Add eggs
and remainder ingredients. Bake at 375 degrees for 10 – 12 minutes.

BREADS
PUMPKIN BANANA BREAD

1 c pumpkin, cooked	½ c banana
1 c brown sugar	½ c butter
3 eggs	2 1/2 c flour
1 t baking powder	1 t cinnamon
½ t ginger	¼ t salt
1 1/2 c nuts, chopped	

Mix pumpkin, banana, sugar and butter well. Beat in eggs. In medium bowl combine flour, baking powder, cinnamon, ginger and salt. Then add the pumpkin mixture, stir in nuts. Pour into 2 greased loaf pans 7 ½ x 3 1/2 x2 Bake in preheated oven of 450 degrees for 50-60 minutes. Remove and cool completely before serving.

Ethel Bell

HONEY BRAN ROLLS

½ c. oil	1 c lukewarm water
1 c boiling water	1 pkg. yeast
1c. bran	2 c w/w flour
2/3 c. honey	1 ½ t salt
2-3 c unbleached white	flour

Combine oil, boiling water, bran, honey and salt. Stirring to blend, cool to lukewarm. Add yeast which has been softened in lukewarm water. Add flour gradually to make soft dough. Knead until smooth and satiny. Let rise to double in bulk about 1 ½ hrs.

Oil hands well (dough will be sticky) form dough into little balls. Drop into a oiled muffin pan or on a baking sheet, and allow to rise about 35-45 minutes. Bake for 25 -40 minutes until nicely browned.

Bobbie Drummond

BREADS
Fresh Fruit Oat Muffin

1 c w/w flour	1 c oats
½ c wheat bran	½ c brown sugar
1 t salt	¼ c butter
1 ½ c buttermilk	2 eggs
3 c. peaches	3. T Orange Juice
1 ½ t. cinnamon.	

Combine all ingredients and spoon into a prepared muffin pan. Bake 400 degrees for 20 minutes.

Serves: 20   Ethel Bell

Banana Nut Bread

½ c. butter	1 1/3 c sugar
2 T. milk	3 eggs
1 ¾ c. flour	1 t. salt
½ t. baking powder	

1t . nutmeg 1 c nuts, chopped

Mashed Bananas (2)

Cream together butter and sugar, add bananas and milk, mixing well. Then fold in nuts. Bake at 350 degree for 45 minutes or until tested done.

Ethel Bell

Excellent when served with cream cheese or any other spread.

BREADS

Potato Rolls

2 T dry active yeast	½ c warm water
2 c hot water	2 c mashed potato
3 T honey	1T salt
2 T oil	½ c wheat germ
¼ soy flour	1 c wheat flour

3T gluten (optional) 4 c unbleached flour

Soften yeast in ½ c warm water. Combine hot water, mashed potatoes, honey, salt and oil. When warm add wheat germ, soy flour, whole wheat flour and gluten. Stir in yeast and add remaining flour to make moderately stiff dough. Turn out on a lightly floured surface. Knead until smooth and satiny. Shape dough into a ball and place in lightly oiled bowl. Cover and let rise for 1 ½ hours. Shape into rolls and let rise again for 40 minutes. Bake at 350 degrees for 25-35 minutes.

Bobbie Drummond

Dips
Spinach Dip
1 (10oz.) pkg. frozen spinach, thawed and drained

1 c. soy mayonnaise

1 c. sour cream

1 onion, chopped

1 can water chestnuts, sliced

1 pkg. *Knorr vegetable soup mix

Mix together all ingredients and let stand in refrigerator at least 24 hours serve with a buttery cracker.

Yield: 3 cups   Jane Spann

Cucumber Onion Dip
1 ½ c. cucumber, shredded and drained

1 c. sour cream

½ c. Miracle Whip salad dressing

½ c. onions, chopped

¼ t salt

¼ t. McCormick All –Purpose seasoning

Dash of Cayenne pepper

Combine all ingredients, mix well, Chill, Serve with raw vegetables.

Yield: 1 cup   Martha Bethea

Cucumber Cheese Dip

8 oz. cream cheese, softened

2 T. whipping cream

1/3 c. minced cucumber

1 t. onion, grated

Salt to taste

¼ t. cumin, ground

¼ t. McCormick All purpose seasoning

Combine cream cheese and whipping cream. Beat on medium speed of mixer for 2 minutes until smooth. Stir in remaining ingredients. Chill, serve with raw vegetables.

Yield: 2 cups   Martha Bethea

Guacamole Dip

soft ripe avocados, mashed

¼ c. soy mayonnaise

1 T. lemon juice

1 T. grated onions

1 large tomato

¼ c McCormick seasoning

Salt to taste

Peel, drain and finely chop tomato. Combine all ingredients. Cover tightly and chill. Serve with tortilla chips, or raw veggies.

Yield: 2 cups   Martha Bethea

Dips

Cucumber Onion Dip

1 ½ c. shredded cucumber, well drained

1 c. sour cream

½ c. Miracle Whip salad dressing

½ c. chopped onion

½ t. salt   Dash of pepper

Combine all ingredients. Mix well. Chill, serve with raw vegetables.

Serves: 4-6   Rhonda C. Edwards

Cucumber Cheese Dip

8oz. cream cheese, softened

2 T. whipping cream

1/2c minced cucumber

1 t. onion

½ t. salt

½ t. cumin, ground

Combine all ingredients and beat in mixer for 2 minutes. Serve with vegetables.

Yield: 1 2/3 cups   Martha Bethea

Dips

Pecan Cheese Log

1 pkg.(8oz) cream cheese, softened

1 c. grated Swiss cheese

1 c. crumbled blue cheese

Season to taste,   ¼ c chopped pecans

Blend all ingredients except pecans

Chill until firm. Shape into log and roll in the pecans. Wrap with plastic wrap and chill. Serve with crackers.

Betty G. Perry

Cream Cheese Spread

1 pkg.(3 oz) cream cheese

1 t. onion juice

½ c. olives (mushrooms if desired)

Dash of salt

Combine all ingredients and serve with crackers.

Betty G. Perry

Smoky Cheese Rolls

1 (8z) pkg. Worthington Vegetarian Entrée', smoked beef style

1 lb. cheddar cheese, Tooth picks

Cut cheese into sticks, and then roll 1 slice of

Entrée' around cheese sticks, securing with toothpicks. Broil until cheese is soft about ½ minute. Addition of an olive per toothpick is festive.

Soups

Grandma's "Beefy" Soup

1roll beef style, cut in chunks

1 onion, chopped

2qts. Water

4T. beef- style granules

1 bag hash brown potatoes

4 cloves garlic, minced

Salt and pepper to taste

3 T. olive oil

Combine the water and beef-style granules into a rolling boil. Then add remainder of ingredients and cook for 15 minutes.

Serves: 4-6

"Sausage Stew"

1can broth	1c water
1bay leaf	1 lg. onion, quarters
6 carrots, julienne,	Sage, thyme, chopped
2 stalks celery, diced	Salt & pepper
1 pkg. frozen hash browns potatoes	
1 T. flour	3T. Olive oil
1 roll *Prosage cubed	
3T. olive oil	

Combine all ingredients, bring to a boil and simmer for 25 minutes.   Mary Smith

Spinach Potato Soup

T butter,   1 c leeks, sliced

1½ lbs potatoes, cubed

cans broth,   4 c. spinach chopped

1t. lemon juice

3T. chicken-style broth

In large pot, place all ingredients brining to a boil and simmer for 30 minutes.

Serve: 7

Cream of Vegetables Soup

2 medium carrots, cut

med potatoes, cubed

1 stalk celery, diced

1 onion, diced

T chicken-style granules

3 c. water

2 c milk

Combine all ingredients and cook for 30 minutes until vegetables are tender. Whiz half of mixture in blender at a time and return to pot.

Serves: 6   Florine Tyler

Broccoli Soup

2 T onions, chopped	2 t butter
3 T flour	1 ½ t salt
3 c. milk	3 c chi-style broth
1 pkg. broccoli	2 c carrots, sliced
Salt and pepper	

In large sauce pan sauté' onion in butter with a whisk stir in flour, salt and milk. Add broth, bring to a boil. Add broccoli and carrots, cook over low heat, stirring occasionally for 25 minutes. Add seasonings to taste. Serve hot.

Yield: 2 quarts.

Cheesy Chicken Chowder

8 T butter	½ c flour
c milk	1 t salt
2 c *Fri- chick	
2 c carrots, shredded	
½ c onion, chopped	
c chicken style broth	
1 c corn, fresh or frozen	
1 teaspoon Worcestershire sauce	
8 ounce cheddar cheese, shredded	

Melt butter in a skillet. Add carrots and onion; sauté until tender. Blend in flour. Add broth and milk. Cook and stir until thick and smooth. Add remaining ingredients and stir until cheese is melted.   Ethel Bell

CHICKEN LEMON SOUP

1 Quart chicken broth

¼ c uncooked rice

Pinch of mace or nutmeg

3egg yolks

Juice of 1 lemon

Seasoning to taste

Place broth, rice and mace in a large saucepan. Cover, and simmer 25- 30 minutes until rice is tender. Beat yolks with lemon juice. Spoon a little hot broth into the egg mixture; return to pan and heat over lowest heat for 1 – 2 minutes, stirring constantly, until no taste of raw egg remains. Do not boil. Season with salt and pepper to taste.   Ethel Bell

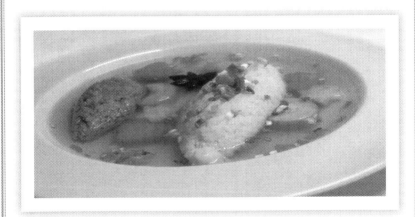

STEWS – SOUPS

Lentil Soup

½ lb dry lentils

2T. olive oil

5 slices *Morningstar Farm vegetarian bacon strips

small onion, chopped

1 stalk celery, chopped

1 clove garlic, minced

3 small carrots, diced

McCormick All-Purpose seasoning to taste

Salt to taste

6 c. water

2 t McKay's Chicken Style seasoning

Salt and rinse lentils. In a medium saucepan, heat oil. Stir in vegetarian bacon, onion, celery, carrots, and garlic.

Add lentils and remaining ingredients. Bring to a boil. Reduce heat; cover, and simmer until lentils are tender and soup get thick. Add more hot water if necessary.

Serves: 4-6   Jessie White

Ramen Noodles Chicken Soup

2pkg. ramen noodles

4c McKay's Style Chicken Broth

1 c Onion, chopped

¼ c. celery, chopped

1 tomato, chopped

Simmer broth, onion, and celery in medium saucepan. Break noodles into small pieces. Place in broth. Continue to simmer until done. Serve in deep bowls topped with topped with tomato.

                         Ethel Bell

SAVORY TOMATO-SPINACH SOUP

*PKG. Morningstar Farm Crumbles

4cups beef style broth

1/4 teaspoon salt

4 potatoes, cubed

3 green onions sliced

1 1/2 pound fresh spinach, washed and coarsely chopped

4 tomatoes, peeled and cut into wedges

¼ teaspoon nutmeg

Combine bouillon, salt, potatoes and onions; cover, cook 20 minutes. To serve: sprinkle each serving lightly with nutmeg

Betty G. Perry

STEWS – SOUPS
TOTILLA SOUP

1 jar Ortega Mild Green Chile Salsa

1 Chicken Style Broth, (2 cups)

1 small zucchini, halved and sliced

1 cup cooked garbanzo beans

2 tablespoons Ortega diced Jalapenos

Tortilla chips, coarsely broken

¾ cup shredded Monterey jack cheese

In saucepan, combine first 5 ingredients; simmer 5-7 minutes. Arrange a shallow layer of chips in serving bowls. Ladle in soup; top with cheese, serve immediately.

Betty G. Perry

CORN CHEESE SOUP

4T butter

3 c. cubed and cooked   potatoes

T. *Baco- chips

1 onion, diced   3 c milk

2 cans corn   1 ½ c yellow cheese

Seasonings

Melt butter and lightly sauté' onion, then add *Baco-chips and all ingredients and heat thoroughly. Yields approximately 2 ½ quarts

Serves 4-6   Annie Flowers

CREAM OF CORN SOUP

2 1/2 cream corn   1 ½ t salt

1 c milk   ½ t. onion

3 T butter   3 c. milk or cream

3 T. flour   dash of nutmeg

Combine corn and milk. Melt butter in skillet and add flour, salt and onion. Stir in corn and 3 more cups milk. Simmer until piping hot, stirring to prevent sticking. Serve in cups with a dash of nutmeg on top.

STEWS – SOUPS
SQUASH SOUP

3 yellow squash	3 zucchini squash
1 onion, diced	1 pepper, diced
3 cloves garlic	24 oz V 8 vegetable
Seasonings	juice
3T chicken –style	
broth	¼ c olive oil
2 c Hash brown potatoes	

Sauté onions, peppers and garlic in oil. Whiz the squash in blender, then combine all ingredients in large pot, simmer for 30 to 45 minutes. Serve with cornbread.

Betty G. Perry

This soup is also excellent as a gravy or sauce.

Easy Squash Soup

med squash, cooked& mashed

envelopes onion soup mix

3 c water or broth

2 cloves, garlic, minced

1 envelope favorite rice or potato dish

Combine all ingredients and cook for 15-20 minutes.

GREEN PLANTAIN SOUP

4c McKay's Chicken Style seasoning broth

2 garlic cloves, minced

¼ c. vegetable oil

3green plantains, peeled and sliced

McCormick All-Purpose seasoning to taste

Salt to taste

Fry the plantains until tender and brown on both sides in the oil. Combine other ingredients in a pot and bring to a boil then add the plantains, stir often, cook for about 15 minutes. Season to taste.

Serves: 4-6   Martha Bethea

Helpful hint: to peel a green plantain, take a small knife and slit through the skin from tip in several places. Then peel each strip of the fruit.

STEWS – SOUPS

Egg Drop Noodle Soup

20 oz chick broth

3 c water

3 1 ½ c fine noodles, uncooked

2 eggs, beaten

2 t. parsley, chopped

3 T butter

Bring broth and water to a boil; add noodles, stirring, cook 8 minutes. Reduce heat to low, stir in eggs, simmer 3 minutes longer. Remove from heat and stir in parsley and butter.

Serves: 4

EZ Cream of Broccoli Soup

2 pkg. broccolis, chopped, cooked

2 cans cream of mushroom soup

2 2/3 c milk

3T butter

½ t tarragon

Seasonings

Combine all ingredients and simmer over low heat until thoroughly heated.

Serves: 8

Golden Pumpkin Soup

1 c. onion, chopped

½ c celery, chopped

2 T butter

2 c broth

1 ½ c mushrooms, sliced

½ c. rice, uncooked

Seasonings

¼ t curry powder

¼ t tarragon

1 can pumpkin, mashed

2 t butter

Sauté' vegetables in large stockpot add remaining ingredients and simmer 30-40 minutes.

Maude van Putten

EZ Cream of Potato Soup

2 c. cubed white potatoes

2 cans cream of mushroom soup

2/ 2/3 c. milk

3 T butter

½ t tarragon

Seasonings

Combine all ingredients and simmer on low for 30 minutes.

STEWS – SOUPS
Italian Rice and Pea soup

1/3 c. olive oil

1 Morningstar Farms Breakfast Strip, chopped

1 slice Wham*, chopped

1 sm. Onion, chopped

1 pkg. frozen peas

1 qt broth or water

½ c rice, uncooked

Seasonings

3 T parmesan cheese

Sauté onion, breakfast strip and Wham slice until light brown. Add peas and cook for 5 minutes. Add liquid and bring to a boil. Add rice, seasonings and cheese, cook until rice is done.

Creamy Carrot Soup

2 T butter	2 c broth
1 c milk	1 t salt
¼ t nutmeg	1/8 t. pepper
¼ c onions and celery, chopped	
2 c. carrots, pureed	

Melt butter add onion and celery sauté until tender. Add carrots, milk nutmeg and pepper and simmer 5-10 minutes. Do not boil.

Chick a Leek Soup

1 dozen leeks cut in ½ "long pieces

2 stalks celery, chopped

1 carrot, chopped

1 c Fri-Chiks*, diced

Seasonings

1 egg yolk

1 oz. butter

Trim vegetables in the butter, when brown add 1 qt. broth and the *Fri-chik. Add seasonings and simmer for 1 hour. Add egg yolk and stir well.

Serves: 4

Maine Corn Chowder

5 slices Breakfast strips	¼ c olive oil
2 med. Onions, sliced	Salt & pepper
3c. potatoes, diced	2 c water
1 can cream style corn	2 c. milk

Sauté breakfast strips in oil with onions, then add potatoes, water salt and pepper. Bring to a boil about 15 minutes until potatoes are done. Add corn and milk. Heat thoroughly. Garnish with crumbled Strips.

Serves: 9

STEWS – SOUPS

Lentil Soup

½ lb dry lentils	1 clove garlic, minced
2 T olive oil	1 pkg. onion soup mix
1 onion, chopped	r c. water
1 stalk celery,	salt and pepper
	Chopped

Heat oil and stir in celery, garlic and onion. Add remaining ingredients and bring to boil, reduce heat and simmer until lentils are tender, and soup gets thick.

Serve: 4   Martha Bethea

PUMPKIN SOUP

1 Med. Pumpkin, chopped	6 c water
Salt and pepper	¼ c. olive oil
2 T chicken style broth	2 cloves garlic
2 lg. potatoes, diced	
1 c. onion, peppers and celery, diced	

Cook pumpkin and potatoes until tender. Sauté' onion, pepper and celery in oil, then combine all ingredients and let simmer for 30 minutes.

TEXAS CHILI

3 T oil   ½ c onion, diced

1/3 c green pepper, chopped

1/3 c red pepper, chopped

1 T chili powder   ½ t salt

1 16 oz. can pinto beans

½ t cayenne pepper

1 16 oz can tomato paste

1 16 oz can diced tomatoes

1 pkg. Morningstar Farm Cumbers

Saute' vegetables, then combine all ingredients bring to a boil and simmer for 15 minutes.

Martha Bethea

CAULIFLOWER CHEESE SOUP

1 head cauliflower   1 can broth

2 t. onion, minced   3 c milk

2 T butter   2 T. flour

Seasonings   2c cheese, grated

Break cauliflower into small pieces and cook. Sauté' onion in butter, blend in flour and seasonings and stir in broth and milk. Combine all ingredients and boil for 30 minutes.

STEWS – SOUPS

Veggie Stew

4T. flour

1 t. salt

1can tomato soup

2c. water, + chop lets* juice

3stalks celery, chopped

1 lg. onion, chopped

1 bay leaf

1 c. peas

4 carrots, diced

2 c. Chop lets*, diced

Combine salt, flour and Choplets* and brown in oil. In large pot combine all ingredients except peas and simmer for 45 minutes, covered. Adding water if needed. Add peas and cook for 15 minutes more. Serve as a stew or use pastry shells and make a pot pie.

Annie Flowers

Corn Chowder

5 slices *Morningstar Breakfast Strips

2 onions, diced

2 c water

1 can cream corn

¼ c. olive oil

3 c. potatoes, sliced

seasonings

2 c milk

Sauté' breakfast strips in oil. Boil potatoes and seasonings until tender. Combine all ingredients and simmer for 15 minutes.

Serve: 9   Annie Flowers

Classic Chili

2 bell peppers (yellow, red or green cut into pieces)
1 can diced tomatoes
2 cloves garlic, minced   2 tsp oil
1 can black beans   1 can chili beans
1 onion, chopped   1 can green chilies,
1T chili powder   ½ t. ground cumin
1 pkg.* Morning Star Crumbles

Cook and stir peppers, onion, and garlic with oil in large saucepan on medium heat for 3 minutes. Add remaining ingredients; bring to a boil and reduce heat. Simmer 30 minutes, stirring occasionally. Serve with sour cream or other favorite toppings.
Serves: 8   Pastor Perry

SAUCES—GRAVIES

Cashew-Pimiento sauce

1 c. water   ½ c cashews
½ c yeast flakes   1/3 c pimiento
1 t. salt   1 t. onion powder
¼ t. garlic powder   ¼ c lemon juice

Blend smooth all ingredients except lemon juice. When the mixture is smooth add the juice. Chilling will make sauce slightly thicker.
                              Rudene Morton

Soy Mayonnaise

½ c soymilk powder   ¾ c water
¾ t. salt   1/8 t. garlic powder
1 ½ t. onion powder   ¼ c. oil
2 T. lemon juice

Blend ingredients except lemon juice and oil. Then add slowly add oil and lemon juice.
                              Rudene Morton

Tender-Bits* Sandwich Filling

2 c Tender-Bits* with liquid (or other vegan-meat)

¼ c chopped parsley

2 T mayo

1 onion, chopped

½ c celery, chopped

¼ c pickle relish

Blend or process the meat and liquid, add remaining ingredients and spread over bread or crackers.

Annie Flowers

Chicken Style Seasoning

½ nutritional yeast flakes

1/8 t oregano

1 t. turmeric

1 T. onion powder

1 T parsley

1/8 t basil

2 t. garlic powder

½ t. sage

½ t. sea salt

Blend and store in a sealed container in refrigerator.

Bobbie Drummond

Thousand Island dressing

1 c mayo

2 T dice pimentos

1/8 t dill seed

¼ c chives, chopped

2 t. tomato juice

¼ c diced olives

¼ c onion, diced

¼ c parsley, chopped

1 t. paprika

Mix all ingredients together. If too thick add a little juice.

Bobbie Drummond

Nutty Sandwich Spread

1 can *Nuteena	1 t. salt
¼ c celery	2 t onion, grated
¼ c pickle relish	1 c. mayo

Combine all ingredients.

Annie Flowers

SAUCES

Lemon Butter

1/3 c oleo or butter	¼ t. salt
2 T lemon juice	1T parsley, chopped

Combine all ingredients and heat and stir.
Serve over spinach, potatoes, etc.

Betty G. Perry

Herbed Butter

1 sm. container soft margarine or butter
1 t parsley
3 cloves garlic, minced
Seasoning salt

Sauté' garlic until tender, stir remaining ingredients into the container. Serve on toast or any vegetable.

Betty G. Perry

Avocado Dressing

2 avocados, peeled	1 carton yogurt
½ c mayo	¼ c onion, diced
2 T lemon juice	1 t sugar
½ t. garlic salt	Tabasco, dash

Combine all in blender until smooth.

Cashew Nut Butter

2c cashews, toasted   ¼ c olive oil

Pinch sugar   dash of salt

Blend and serve

BUTTERMILK HERB DRESSING

1 c. buttermilk   salt

1 t. chives, chervil & watercress, chopped

½ t tarragon   ¼ t. mustard

Blend and serve.

AVOCADO DRESSING

2 avocados   8oz carton yogurt

½ c mayo   ¼ c lemon juice

1 T honey   ½ t. garlic salt

½ t. salt   Tabasco, dash

All ingredients in blender until smooth and pureed. Store covered in refrigerator.

Yield: 2 ½ cups

APPETIZERS

English muffin Snacks

½ c. mayo

1 can olives, chopped   ½ t. curry powder

½ c green onions, chopped

1 1/2c cheese, grated

6 split English muffins

Mix all ingredients and spread on muffins. Broil until bubbly. Quarter and serve.

Mushrooms Pastries

1 can refrigerated bread dough

½ pkg. *Crumbles

1 can cream of mushroom soup

1 can sliced mushrooms, drained

2 T. onion

2 T. Worcestershire sauce

Place all ingredients except bread dough in a saucepan and heat for 3 minutes., On cutting board, flatten each piece of bread dough and spoon the Crumbles* mixture into the center. Pull the dough edges to the center tightly to seal the filling inside. Place buns smooth side up on greased baking sheet. With a sharp knife make a cut on top of each bun for steam escape. Bake at 375 degrees for 35 minutes or until browned.

Open-Faced Egg and Cheese Sandwiches

1 T. butter	2 T. onions, chopped
2 T. green pepper	6 eggs, beaten
1/3 c milk	salt & pepper
6 1oz slices American cheese	
1 T. butter	
6 English muffins halves	

Melt butter in frying pan; sauté' onion and green pepper. Combine eggs, milk, salt and pepper and pour over onions, stirring until eggs are set.

Divide eggs into 6 portions. Spread toasted muffin halves with butter and top with egg mixture followed with 1 slice of cheese. Broil until cheese is slightly browned about 5 minutes.

Lime Salad

1 3 oz pkg. lime gelatin	1 c. hot water
1 c pineapple juice	2T vinegar
3 slices pineapple, diced	
1 pimento, chopped	1 orange, sectioned
½ c celery, diced	½ t salt

Dissolve gelatin in hot water. Add pineapple juice and remaining ingredients. Pour into molds, refrigerate. Serve on curly endive greens.

CURRY DIP

1 c mayo   1T onion, minced
½ t curry powder
Salt and pepper

Combine all ingredients, chill; serve with raw veggies.

APPETIZERS

Spiced Nuts

4 c pecans or walnuts
1 c sugar
1 T cinnamon
½ t salt
1 egg white
1 T water

Put nuts in large bowl; set aside. Mix sugar, Cinnamon and salt in small bowl. In another bowl, beat egg white and water until almost stiff; add to nuts and stir until nuts are well coated. Add sugar mixture and stir. Grease cookie sheet, pour in nuts, and bake in 300 degree oven for 30 minutes, stirring after 15 minutes. When cool separate nuts.

VEGETABLE-ROMA

1 8oz pkg. cream cheese
3 T prepared Roma* cold
1 T carrot, parsley and onion, chopped
Salt and pepper
½ t Worcestershire sauce

Combine cream cheese and Roma until smooth. Stir in remaining ingredients and blend well. Chill. Serve with raw veggies.

CHILI PEPPER DIP

1 can cream of celery soup

1 can green chilies, chopped

1 c cheddar cheese, grated

2 t. onion, minced

Combine all ingredients in a saucepan, stir over low heat to melt the cheese. Serve with chips.

Marshmallow fruit dip

1 pkg. cream cheese

13 oz jar marshmallow crème

½ t ginger

2 T grated orange rind

Dash nutmeg

Pineapple juice

Red and green apples

Combine all ingredients except apples. Core the apples and serve with dip.

APPETIZERS
Pineapple Cheese Spread

1 8oz pkg. cream cheese

1 can crushed pineapple, drained

½ c. pecans, chopped

Beat cheese until light and fluffy, then combine all ingredients and mix well.

CHEESE PUFFS-WICHES

¼ c margarine

1 T pimento

10 slices bread

1 egg

1 jar cheese spread

Trim bread and cut into 4 squares. Combine remaining ingredients together and spread the mixture over the bread then place in the 350 degree oven until slightly browned and puffed.

Seasoned croutons

1 Loaf day old bread, cubed

1 T. parsley

1 T garlic powder

1 stick butter, melted

In small bowl place the herbs and melted butter, stir well. Place the bread cubes on the baking sheet and drizzle with the butter mixture. Bake at 350 degrees for 5-7 minutes, stirring as needed. Delicious with salads.

*BIG FRANKS SPREAD

1 can Big Franks*, mashed

½ c pickle relish

Cayenne pepper

½ c black olives, chopped

10 slices bread

1/2c onion, chopped

¾ c mayo

¼ c mustard

Mix all ingredients except bread. Spread mixture on 5 slices of bread, using the second slice to complete the sandwich. Cut each sandwich into 4 tiny sandwiches. Also excellent when used on crackers.

CONEY ISLAND HOT DOGS

1 #2 can chili con carne	1t. mustard
1 6oz can tomato paste	½ t salt
8 *Big Franks	8 frankfurter rolls

1 T. oiMix chili, tomato paste, mustard and salt in a saucepan. Heat thoroughly. In another pan place the oil and the Big Franks after they have been split down the center. Split the rolls down the center, toast. Place a Big Frank in each roll and a generous amount of chili to cover.

Serves: 8

HINTS !!
Your fruit salads will look perfect when you use an egg slicer too make perfect slices of strawberries, kiwis or bananas.

APPETIZERS

Teenage Submarine

1 pkg. *Wham, cubed	½ lb cheese, cubed
1/3 c sliced scallions	2 boiled eggs, sliced
½ c olives, sliced	3 T mayo
½ c chili sauce	12 frankfurter rolls

Preheat oven to 400 degrees. Combine first 7 ingredients in a bowl. Mix well. Spread mixture on Frankfurter rolls. Wrap each roll in aluminum foil, twisting ends securely. Bake for 10 minutes.

Serves: 4-6

MEXICAN-STYLE BURGERS

1 pkg. *Crumbles	2 t. onion, minced
¾ t oregano, cumin	salt & pepper
4 taco shells	1 tomato, sliced
1 c shredded lettuce	salsa

In large bowl combine Crumbles, onion, oregano, cumin, salt and pepper, mixing thoroughly. Divide the mixture in to 4 oval shape patties. Broil, turning once. Arrange the lettuce, tomato slices with a grilled burger in each taco shell. Top each with ¼ c lettuce and salsa.
Serves: 4

Potato Kisses

3 c water	salt & Pepper
1 lb potatoes, mashed	2 T butter
½ c Swiss cheese, shredded	
1 egg	4 T half & half cream
1 T parsley flakes	

Grease a baking sheet and set aside, preheat oven to 350 degrees. Combine all ingredients well and place into a pastry bag with a star tip. Pipe in the mounds of potatoes on a baking sheet. Bake in oven for 20-25 minutes or until lightly browned.
Serves: 4

Spinach Mashed Potatoes

6-8 lg. potatoes, mashed	¾ sour cream
1 stick butter	salt & pepper
2 T dried chives	¼ t. dill leaves
1 10oz pkg. spinach, cooked	
1 c. shredded cheese	

Combine all ingredients and beat with mixer until light and fluffy. Place in casserole and bake at 400 degrees for 20 minutes.

APPETIZERS
FESTIVE POTATO WEDGES

2 T butter, melted

3 med. Potatoes, unpeeled

1 T Parmesan cheese

1 T parsley flakes

1 t. dry salad dressing mix

Salt & Pepper

Cut potatoes into quarters or wedges. Combine cheese, dry salad mix, parsley flakes in a small dish and sprinkle over potatoes. Cover with plastic wrap and microwave on high for 8-10 minutes or until tender.

Serves: 6

SUNSHINE SWEET POTATOE BALLS

¼ c butter, melted   ¼ c. milk

2 T sugar   salt & pepper

4 c sweet potatoes, cooked and mashed

18-20 miniature marshmallows

3 c *Kellogg's Corn Flakes, crushed

Combine all ingredients except marshmallows and corn flakes. Form into 2 inch balls with a marshmallow center and then roll into the corn flake crumbs. Place in a 9x12x3/4 baking dish and bake for 25-35 minutes.

Yield: 18-20 balls

PICKLED BEETS

2 cans sliced beets	½ c. sugar
1 cinnamon stick	allspice, dash
1 sm. Onion, sliced	vinegar

Combine all ingredients into a large bowl, stir and cover then chill at least 1 hour, enjoy.

Serves: 6-8   Betty G. Perry

BLACK BEAN SALAD

2 T. orange juice	2 T. lemon juice
2 t. olive oil	½ t. salt
½ t. ground cumin	½ t. hot sauce
1 can black beans, drained	
1 c. long grain rice, cooked	
3 plum tomatoes, chopped	
½ red onion, chopped	
½ green pepper, chopped	
2 green onions, sliced	
1 celery rib, diced	

Combine all ingredients together in a large bowl toss gently to coat. Cover and chill for 1 hour.

Serves: 6-8

Bobbie Drummond

APPETIZERS
Four Bean Salad

1 c. kidney beans	½ c. salad oil
1 c. green beans	½ c. lemon juice
1 c. wax beans	1/3 c sugar
1 chick peas	1 onion, chopped
1 stalk celery, chopped	

Drain beans. Mix in other ingredients and mix well. For best results make a day ahead of use. Refrigerate.

Serves: 6-8   Sylvia Bartholomew

WALDORF SALAD

6 apples, peeled and diced

1 c. raisins

Red and green grapes

Mayonnaise

Walnuts if desired

Combine all ingredients and chill

Serves: 6-8   Mary Alford

MINCED OLIVE DIP

1 pt. sour cream	2 t. onion juice

1 can ripe olives, chopped

1 t. *McCormick All Purpose seasoning Salt to taste

Drain olives and combine with sour cream and seasonings. Let stand at least ½ hr. before serving. Serve with chips.

Yield: 3 cups

CUCUMBER SUPREME

2 med. Cucumbers

1 lg. onion, sliced and separated

1 c 7 buttermilk recipe dressing

Green onion tops, chopped.

Peel and slice cucumbers and onions. In a bowl put salad dressing and green onion tops, stir in cucumbers and onion.

Betty G. Perry

GLAZED CARROTS

2 c sliced carrots	½ c sugar
2 T cornstarch	nutmegs

1 c frozen orange juice

Cook and drain carrots. Mix remaining ingredients, cook until thick. Pour sauce over carrots and let stand.

APPETIZERS
PINEAPPLE PUDDING

1 c. sugar   6 T. flour

2 c sharp cheese, grated

2 cans pineapple chunks

1 sleeve *Ritz crackers

1 stick butter, melted

Preheat oven to 350 degrees and grease a casserole dish. In large bowl stir together sugar, flour and cheese then add the drained pineapple chunks; spread the mixture into casserole. In separate bowl combine the crumbs, pineapple juice and butter, stirring until well blended. Spread this mixture over the first mixture and bake at 350 degrees for 30 minutes, or until golden brown.

Serves: 8

BLACKEYE PEA CROQUET

1 can black-eyed peas   3 T. flour

Thyme, sage, parsley chopped

1 egg   2 T oil

2 cloves, minced   1 onion, chopped

1 bell pepper, chopped   salt & pepper

Cayenne pepper, dash

Blend peas, sauté" pepper and onion then combine all ingredients well. Shape into balls and place on a baking sheet or deep fry until golden. Serve with favorite sauce. ***For variation use***

any beans or peas.

CHICKETTE CORDON BLEU

1 box *Fri-Chik patties

4 slices *Breakfast strips

1 T. oil

1 can cream of cheddar soup

Take Chik patties thawed and slice in half width wise. Take a breakfast strip cut in half and place both halves in the center of each patty. Lay each patty in an oiled casserole dish and pour 1 can of cheddar soup over. Bake in 350 degree oven for 20 minutes.

Serves: 4

ZUCCHINI QUICHE'

3 c zucchini, grated	1 c biscuit mix
½ t season salt	½ c onion, chopped
½ t oregano	2 c. mozzarella cheese
2 T. parsley, chopped	½ c oil
4 eggs	2 cloves garlic, minced

Heat oven to 350 degree. Grease 9x13 inch pan. Mix all ingredients, spread in pan. Bake until golden, about 25 minutes. Slice into small squares. Can be served hot or cold.

How to Eat

Chew food thoroughly. Don't wash food down with liquids. Liquids with meals only hinder digestion. Avoid very hot or very cold liquids, as well as strongly spicy and salty foods. Eat enough to satisfy hunger, Overheating is an enemy of proper mental function and dangerous to your health.

APPETIZERS

CRANBERRY-STRAWBERRY MOLD

2 12 oz. cans frozen apple juice
2 c. fresh cranberries
1 ½ c fresh strawberries
1/2c agar flak

Place in blender 1 can frozen apple juice, the cranberries and strawberries. Blend until smooth. Pour mixture into saucepan and add the second can of apple juice and the agar flakes. Bring to boil, pour into mold and chill.

Rudene Morton

*Chik Pasta Salad

2 c tricolored pasta twists
1 T olive oil
1 T olive oil
1 ½ green bean, cooked
3 c *Fri-Chik, chopped
Salt & pepper to taste
Fresh basil, garnish

2 T pesto sauce
1 tomato, chopped
12 black olives

Cook pasta in salt water for about 12 minutes, drain and rinse. In bowl stir pesto sauce and olive oil. Add tomato and olives, seasoning green beans and chik. Toss gently and transfer to a serving dish, garnish with basil.

Bobbie Drummond

*WHAM SPREAD

1 can *Wham, mashed
¼ c onions, diced
¼ celery, diced
Combine all and serve.

1/4 c relish
¼ c peppers
½ c mayo

CELERY PINWHEELS

1 medium stalk celery

1 (3oz) pkg. cream cheese

2 t. Roquefort cheese

Mayo

Worcestershire sauce

Clean celery and separate branches. Blend together the softened cream cheese with the Roquefort; add mayo and make the consistency spreadable and season with a dash of Worcestershire sauce. Fill the branches of the celery with the cheese mixture, then press branches back together in original form and roll in wax paper and chill overnight in refrigerator. Just before serving cut slice celery crosswise forming pinwheels. Arrange pinwheels on bed of crisp lettuce for serving.

Water is absolutely the best beverage for quenching thirst and the best liquid for cleansing the tissues of the body. Drink 6-8 glasses per day. If you weigh more than 250 lbs an additional glass for every 25 lbs is needed. Always check first with your healthcare provider.

ENTREES'

Tomato, Burger N Beans

1 pkg. *Crumbles   ¼ c. oil

1 c water   1 pkg. sloppy Joe mix

1 can tomato paste   1 can mushroom

2 cans french style green beans

FRENCH *TUNO BAKE

1 med eggplant, sliced   1 tomato, sliced

1 green pepper cut in strips

1 zucchini, sliced   2 t lemon juice

¼ c parsley, chopped   salt & pepper

½ thyme   2 cans *Tuno

1 c mozzarella cheese, shredded

Layer vegetables in buttered casserole. Sprinkle parsley and lemon juice, salt ,pepper, thyme and bake uncovered for 45 minutes in 375 oven. Then spread the *Tuno and sprinkle with cheese and bake for 15 minutes more. Very aromatic and delicious.

SOUTHWEST STUFFED PEPPERS

Nonstick spray	1/2c onions, diced
1 c instant brown rice	1c broth
½ c salsa	1 ½ t cumin
¾ c black beans, drained	½ c corn
3 red or green peppers cut in half	
1/3 c cheese, shredded	

Spray medium saucepan with spray, add onions and cook over medium heat for 1 minute. Add rice, ¾ c broth, salsa and cumin. Cover brings to a boil and simmer for 10 minute. Remove from heat and stir in beans and corn. While rice is cooking, place peppers with remaining broth and microwave for 3-4 minutes. Spoon rice mixture into peppers, top with cheese. Cover and microwave on high for 3-4 minutes. Serve with additional salsa if desired.

Serves: 6

Healthful hint:

When desiring oat or rice flour and it is not available, simply whiz 1 cup of uncooked rice or oats into the blender and you will have the flour.

Entrees

Creamy Meat Gravy

1 c raw cashews	2 c water
1 onion, chopped	
1 c bell pepper, chopped	
1 c mushrooms	
2 cloves garlic, minced	
½ c favorite veggie meat	
*Chicken-style seasoning	
2 t. olive oil	

Blend cashews and water until smooth. Combine with other ingredients and heat until it starts to thicken. Stir often. Serve with roasts, biscuits, potatoes, rice, etc.

Serves: 6   Ethel Bell

ZUCCHINI FRITTATA

1 c biscuit mix	½ t. salt
3 c. zucchini, sliced	½ t oregano
1 onion, chopped	3 cloves garlic, minced
1/3 c oil	½ c oil
½ c parmesan cheese	2 T parsley
4 eggs, beaten	

Mix all ingredients. Spread in an oiled 9x12x2 inch pan and bake at 350 degrees for 35 minutes or until golden brown. Good warm or cold.

Serves: 6   Joann Barnes

BROCCOLI, RICE CASSEROLE

1 c rice, cooked	3 T butter
1 onion, chopped	1 jar cheese spread
1 pkg. broccoli, chopped	½ c. milk
1 can cream of mushroom soup	
1 can water chestnuts sliced	

Combine all ingredients together and place in a shallow casserole dish. Bake covered for 30-40 minutes, then uncover for another 10 minutes.

Serve: 6   Joann Barnes

Gourmet Rice

1 stick butter	1 can broth
1 ½ c rice, uncooked	1 can water
1 onion, chopped	1 can mushrooms
Bell peppers and celery, diced (optional)	

Combine all ingredients in a casserole. Place in oven at 350 degrees for 1 hour. Cover, stir once , bake until firm and brown.

Serves: 6-8   Ethel Bell

ENTREES/ KID APPROVED

Pizza Rice

1 T. oil	½ green pepper, sliced
½ onion, sliced	½ t garlic powder
½ t. pepper	1 ½ t oregano
3 oz veggie *Salami	
1 can tomato sauce	1 ½ instant rice
1 c water	
3 t. parmesan cheese	
1 c mozzarella cheese, grated	

Heat the oil in saucepan then add peppers, onion, garlic powder, pepper and oregano and saute' until onion is transparent. Cut up ½ salami and add to veggies, saute'2 minutes. Add tomato sauce, rice and water and 2 t of parmesan cheese, bring to a boil, cover and remove from heat. Let stand 5 minutes. Pour the mixture in a casserole dish, sprinkle top with mozzarella cheese, the salami and parmesan cheese. Bake in a preheated oven for about 6 minutes, or until cheese has melted.

Serves: 4

HINT!!

Egg shells can be easily removed from hard-boiled eggs if they are quickly rinsed in cold water after they are boiled.

Add a drop of food coloring to the boiling water to help tell the cooked egg from the raw eggs in the refrigerator.

Hot Dog Casserole

2 cans vegetarian beans

1 ½ c water

8 1oz. cheese slices

2 c. instant rice

8* Veggie Links

Mix beans, rice and water bring to a boil and cover, remove from heat. Let stand for 5 minutes. Cut *Links in half lengthwise. Pour rice mixture in casserole dish and line the links on top of the rice. Arrange cheese slices over the top bake at 350 degrees for 15 minutes.

Serves 4-8

MEATBALLS AND RICE

1 can *Tender Rounds

2 c instant rice, cooked

Garlic powder, dash

spaghetti sauce

2 T parsley

¼ c Parmesan cheese

Take prepared rice and place in a medium bowl and combine with cheese, garlic powder and parsley. Place *Tender Rounds in a saucepan and add the spaghetti sauce, heat . Serve meatballs over rice.

Serves: 4

SLOPPY JOES

Nonstick spray

½ pkg. *Crumbles

¼ c green pepper, chopped

¾ c tomato sauce

1 c instant rice

½ c onions, chopped

4 sandwich buns

½ c *BBQ sauce

Add all ingredients except buns and cook over low heat. Cook until hot. Spoon into sandwich buns.   Serves : 4

ENTREES
CUBAN BLACK BEAN AND RICE SALAD

2 ½ c water	1 c rice
3 t olive oil	1/2 t. salt
1 can *Tender Bits	2 cloves garlic, diced
½ c mayo	½ c salsa sauce
½ c cilantro, chopped	½ t. pepper
1 can black beans, drained	
6 green onions with tops, cut into pieces	
1 can green chilies, diced	
Torn spinach leaves	

Bring water to a boil and add rice, 1 T oil and salt. Cover and simmer for 20 minutes. Remove from heat and let stand, chill. Sauté' *Tender bits, beans, green onion and chili. Chill. To serve line each serving bowl with spinach leaves; mound salad onto the leaves.

Serves: 5-7

MUSHROOM FETTUCCINE

8 oz. fettuccine, cooked	¼ c parsley
3 c mushrooms, sliced	¼ c oil
3 t. parmesan cheese	2 t. rosemary
Salt and pepper	1 clove garlic, crushed

Cook and drain fettuccine as directed. Rinse with cold water. Add all ingredients and toss.

Serves: 8

PESTO *CHIK AND RICE

1 t. oil	3 cloves garlic, minced
2 T. flour	¾ c broth
¼ c milk	3 c. brown rice
1/3 c. basil, chopped	
½ c parmesan cheeses	
1 can *Fri-chik	

In medium saucepan, heat olive oil, add garlic for 1 minute. Add flour and cook for 30 seconds, add broth and milk and cook for 1 minute. Stir in rice, basil and cheese. Place into 1 qt casserole. Place *Fri-chiks on top of rice and sprinkle a bit more of parmesan cheese. Cover and bake 10 minutes more or until golden brown.,

Serves: 4

CHEESY* DINNER ROAST & MUSHROOMS

½ c rice	2 T butter
2 T flour	1 c milk
2 oz cheese, grated	2 cans mushrooms
4 slices of *Dinner Roast cut into pieces	

Prepare rice. To make cheese sauce, melt butter and stir in flour. Gradually add milk, stirring often until thicken. Remove heat and stir in cheese. Season with salt and pepper. Sauté' mushrooms in remainder of butter. In a casserole dish, spoon a layer of rice then cover with *Dinner Roast, continue to alternate finishing with rice. Bake at 400 degrees for 15 minutes.

Serves: 4-6

ENTREES

RE-FRIED* SWISS STEAKS

1 can *Swiss Steaks (save gravy)

Flour	sliced onions
Sliced peppers	oil
1 can mushrooms	steak sauce

Take each steak and batter in flour and brown in oil on both sides. Remove steaks from pan and sauté' onions and peppers, add 1 T flour in pan and stir until browned, adding 2 cups water and steak sauce then simmer until thickened. Add mushrooms and steaks. Transfer to a serving dish.

Betty G. Perry

May use any other vegan-meats just as well.

SHEPHERD'S PIE

1 can *Redi-burger	beef style broth
1 can mushrooms	1 stick butter
Mashed potatoes	2 eggs
Seasonings	garlic, minced

1 c. onions, peppers and celery (chopped)

Sauté' vegetables in butter, then brown the *Redi-burger. Combine all ingredients except eggs and potatoes. Pour meat mixture into a oiled casserole dish. Take the potatoes and stir in the eggs then pile potato mixture over the *Redi-burger mixture. Bake in oven for 30 minutes at 350 degrees.

Serves: 8   Martha Bethea

GRAPE-NUTS LOAF

2c. *Grape-Nuts cereal

3 c. milk

2 c. celery, onion chopped

½ c nuts

2 T. flour(wheat)

salt and pepper

1 t. sage/thyme

Combine all ingredients well, and let stand for 20 minutes. Transfer to oiled 2 qt. casserole. Bake uncovered at 350 degrees for 40 minutes until lightly browned. Let stand 5 minutes before serving.

Rudene Morton

HAYSTACKS

Corn chips

shredded lettuce

Shredded cheese

green onions, sliced

Tomatoes, diced

peppers, sliced

Radishes, diced

sour cream

Salsa sauce

1 can pinto beans

Ripe olives, diced

Layer individual salads starting with corn chips.

BBQ KABOBS

1 each green, red, yellow bell peppers cut in chunks.

12 cloves garlic

black olives

Pineapple chunks

cherry tomatoes

12 skewers

BBQ sauce

1 Box* Morningstar Farm Buffalo Wings

Add a portion of each ingredient onto the skewer, then place the skewer in a sprayed oblong baking dish, pour sauce over and bake for 10 minutes.

MEXICAN SALAD

1 onion	4 tomatoes
1 head lettuce	4 oz cheddar, grated
8 oz French dressing	salt & Pepper
2 c corn chips	1 can kidney beans
1/4c oil	2 c *Crumbles

Brown *Crumbles in oil, then add kidney beans and simmer for 10 minutes. Chop onion, tomato and lettuce and place in a large bowl. Toss in cheese and dressing and chips. Mix the *Crumbles mixture to the salad bowl and serve.

HOT *CHIKETTE SALAD

1 roll *Chickette, diced	2 c celery, diced
1 can water chestnuts	½ c mayo
2 T. lemon juice	½ t. salt
2 T grated onion	shredded cheese
Potato chips, crushed	

Mix all ingredients except cheese and chips and pour into greased baking dish. Cover with the cheese. Bake at 350 degree for 15 minutes then cover with potato chips and return to oven for 5-7 minutes.

Serves: 8   Betty G. Perry

MEXICAN RICE

2 c. rice, cooked	1 l. jar salsa
Taco seasoning	1 c. grated cheese
1 T. crushed red peppers	
2 t. oil	

Combine and pour into oiled casserole and bake 350 degrees for 30 minutes.

BEAN SALAD

3 cans kidney beans	1c onions, diced
1 c sweet pickle, diced	2 T cider vinegar
3 hard boiled eggs, diced	3 T sugar

Combine all ingredients, keep refrigerated.

BAJA POTATO SALAD

4 l. potatoes, cooked & cubed

1 onion, diced   1 can green chilies

4 T cilantro, chopped

1 8oz pkg. cream cheese

1 oz canned jalapenos, diced

½ t salt

1 clove garlic, minced

Salt & pepper

Combine together all ingredients.
Serves: 4-6

SWEET POTATO CASSEROLE

2 cans sweet potatoes, mashed

7 T. butter, melted

1 apple, thinly sliced

TOPPING:

¼ c brown sugar, firmly packed

1 T. flour

¼ t. cardamom

1 T cold butter

2 T pecans, chopped

Preheat oven to 350 degrees. In 1 qt. casserole, place sweet potatoes, add butter. In small bowl cut 1 T cold butter into brown sugar, flour and cardamom. Stir in pecans and sprinkle ½ of this mixture over the sweet potatoes. Arrange apple slices on top and sprinkle with remaining mixture. Bake for 35 to 40 minutes or until apples are tender/crisp.

Serves: 6

ENCHILADA CASSEROLE

12 corn tortillas

2 pkg. * Crumbles

2 T. chili powder

1 c cheese, grated

1 can cream of mushroom soup

1 onion, chopped

1 can tomato sauce

½ t. garlic powder

¾ c milk

Brown *Crumbles, garlic and onions. Heat a 9x13 pan and place 6 tortillas. Combine all the ingredients and spread on top of tortillas. Cover with 6 tortillas and shredded cheese. Bake 25 minutes at 350 degrees.

Serve: 8

CROWD PLEASER CASSEROLE

1 20 oz. pkg. broccoli flowerets

1 20 oz pkg. cauliflower flowerets

4 T butter	3 T flour
3 c milk	6 oz. cheddar shredded

1 c Parmesan cheese, grated

Seasonings

3 c chopped *Wham(ham style vegan-meat)

3 c bread crumbs, tossed with 4 t. butter

Cook broccoli and cauliflower underdone, set aside. Melt 4 t butter in a quart saucepan, add flour and blend well. Add milk, stirring constantly until thickened. Add cheese and seasonings. Place veggies in casserole, sprinkle chopped wham over then pour cheese mixture over, then sprinkle bread crumbs over top. Bake uncovered for 30 minutes at 350 degrees.

Serves: 10-12

MACARONI AND CHEESE WITH SOUR CREAM

1 ½ c macaroni, cooked	2/3 c sour cream
2 c cheddar, grated	1/3 c milk

Paprika

Seasoning

Combine all ingredients and mix well. Place into a greased baking dish and bake at 325 degrees for 30 minutes. Sprinkle paprika on top,

Serves: 4

ENTREES
MACARONI HOT DISH

2 c macaroni cooked and warm

1 ½ c cheese, grated	1 ½ c bread crumbs
1 green pepper, diced	1 onion, diced
3 eggs, beaten	2T butter, melted
Seasonings	1 ½ c milk

1 can mushroom soup

Mix all ingredients, except mushroom soup and place in a pan set in hot water. Bake at 350 degrees for 45 minutes. Cut in squares and then pour over heated undiluted mushroom soup.

Serves: 6

GRITS CASSEROLE

1 pkg. *Breakfast patties

½ c green peppers,	1 c onion chopped
1 c grits, uncooked	4 c water or broth
Seasonings	1 c cheese, grated

1 can cream of mushroom or celery soup

Preheat oven to 375 degrees. Crumble and brown breakfast patty, adding peppers, onions and celery. Cook grits in the water or broth. Combine cooked grits and breakfast patties mixture and pour into a 2 quart casserole. Spread soup over the top and sprinkle with the cheese. Bake for 30 minutes.

Serves: 10-12

*CHIK-BROCCOLI BAKE

1 10 OZ. pkg. broccoli cuts
2 c *Fri-Chik, chopped
4 oz. medium noodles, cooked
1 c sour cream
1 can cream of mushroom soup
2 T pimiento, chopped
1 T. onion, minced
Seasonings
½ t. Worcestershire sauce
1 T melted butter
½ c bread crumbs
1 c cheese, grated

Cook broccoli partially. Add butter to breadcrumbs and set aside. Combine chik, sour cream, soup, pimiento, onion, seasonings and Worcestershire sauce. Place noodles in prepared shallow 2 qt baking dish. Sprinkle with 1/3 of the cheese. Add broccoli, sprinkle with ½ of remaining cheese. Pour on the chicken mixture and sprinkle with remainder of cheese and then with the bread crumbs. Bake at 350 degrees for 1 hour.

"BEEFY" CASSEROLE

1 large eggplant, cooked, sliced
1 med onion, chopped
2 T butter
1 pkg. *Morningstar Farms Crumbles
Seasonings to taste
4 slices cheese

Saute' onion in butter until soft, add *Crumbles and seasonings, cook until nicely browned. Place slices of eggplant in a greased baking dish and add Crumbles mixture. Cover with thin slices of cheese. Bake at 400 degrees for 20 minutes or until cheese is melted.

*WHAM & NOODLE CASSEROLE

¼ c margarine	¼ c flour
½ t salt	2 ½ c milk
1 pkg. *Wham cubes(ham-style vegan)	
2 c noodles, cooked	1 t. mustard
¾ c bread crumbs	
2 T melted margarine	
1 can peas and carrots	

Preheat oven to 375 degrees, melt margarine in a skillet. Blend in flour and seasonings, gradually stir in milk. Cook over medium heat, stirring constantly until mixture is smooth and thick. Add *Wham, noodles, mustard, peas and carrots, mix well. Spoon into greased 1 ½ qt. casserole. Combine bread crumbs and margarine, then sprinkle over noodles. Bake 25 minutes.

BAKED RICE WITH HERBS

2 T butter	1 green onion, minced
¼ c parsley, chopped	¼ t thyme
¼ t sage	seasonings
1 c brown rice	2 ½ c broth or water
½ t garlic powder	

Preheat oven to 350 degrees. Place butter into baking dish and sauté' onions. Add all ingredients and cover. Let cook for 45 minutes or until liquid is absorbed and rice is tender.

LADIES LUNCHEON LAYERED DISH

1 c crushed potato chips

4 hard boiled eggs, sliced

1 onion, sliced thin and separated

1/3 c parsley

1 can cream of mushroom soup

¼ c sour cream

¾ c milk

½ t paprika

Spread 1/3 of potato chips in bottom of oiled dish. Cover with 1/3 of eggs slices and 1/3 of onion rings and parsley. Repeat layers.

Combine soup with sour cream, milk and paprika, mixing well, then pour over the layers, cover and bake at 350 degrees for 30 minutes. Remove cover and bake 10 minutes more until golden brown.

ENCHILADA SQUARES

1 pkg. *Morningstar Farms Crumbles

1 c onion, chopped

4 oz can diced chilies

4 eggs

8 oz can tomato sauce

1 can evaporated milk

1 envelope enchilada mix

1 t chili powder

1 c cheese, shredded

½ c black olives, sliced

¼ c oil

Brown *Crumbles and onion in oil. Spread this mixture in a s oiled 10x6x2 inch pan. Sprinkle green chilies over meat mixture. Beat egg, tomato sauce, evaporated milk and enchilada sauce and olives. Spread this over the top. Bake 350 degrees for 25 minutes, then sprinkle the cheese and bake 5 minutes more. Set 10 minutes before cutting.

Entrees

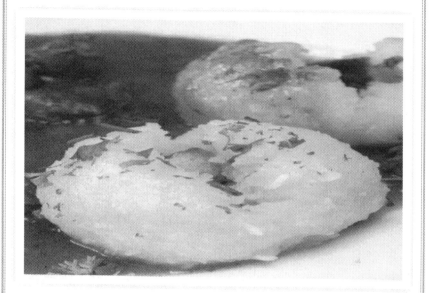

What is a meal without a nice entrée?

*CHIK ALMOND CASSEROLE

5C *Fri-Chik, diced	½ c sour cream
2 c celery, diced	½ c mayo
3 c rice, cooked	2 T onion, chopped
1 can water chestnuts, sliced	
2 cans mushroom soup	2 T lemon juice
Seasoning	1c almonds, sliced

Combine above ingredients and place in a buttered 9x13 baking dish.

TOPPING:

½ c almonds, sliced

3 c corn flake crumbs

2/3 c butter

Combine the above and sprinkle on top of casserole. Bake at 350 degrees for 35-45 minutes.

BREAKFAST SANDWICH

4 eggs hard boil and finely chopped

4 *Morningstar Breakfast strips, brown

& chopped

¼ c mayo	1 c. cheese grated
1 t tarragon	1 ¼ t mustard
8 slices whole wheat bread	

Mix together all ingredients except bread. Spread mixture evenly between 8 slices of bread forming 4 sandwiches. Spread melted butter on outside surfaces of sandwiches. Brown on both sides in heavy skillet.

Serves: 4

ENTREES
VEGETABLE CAKE
Base:

2 T vegetable oil

4 large potatoes, thinly sliced

TOPPING:

1 can *Fri-Chik, diced

1 T vegetables oil

1 leek, chopped

1 zucchini, grated

1 carrot, grated

1 red pepper, diced

salt & pepper

2 eggs, beaten

8 oz. cheese, shredded

2 T. parsley, chopped

1 green pepper, diced

Grease an 8 inch spring form cake pan. Make the base by heating the base in oil in frying pan until brown. Then arrange them on the bottom of the cake pan.

In a skillet sauté' the leeks for 2-3 minutes, add the remaining vegetables, cooking for 5-7 minutes, now add *Fri-chik, season. Beat together the cheese and eggs and combine with the vegetable mixture; spoon this mixture over the potato base. Cook in a preheated oven at 375 degrees for 20-25 minutes until cake is set. Remove from pan and serve.

Serves: 4   Mary Smith

SOUPER CHIK CASSEROLE

2 cups *Fri-chik, diced

1 (16oz) bag frozen vegetables

1 can mushroom soup

1 can French fried onion rings

1/3 c sour cream

¼ t salt

¼ t. pepper

Combine all ingredients except the cheese and onions. In casserole dish pour ½ vegetables and add ½ cheese and ½ onions and repeat. Bake uncovered for 25 minutes at 350 degrees.

STEAK POTATO CASSEROLE

1(32OZ) HASH BROWN POTATOES, FROZEN

½ c butter, melted	8oz cheese, shredded
1 c onions, chopped	1 pt. sour cream
1 can mushroom soup	salt & pepper
½ t garlic powder	1 c corn flakes
¼ c melted margarine	

Partially defrost potatoes, mix potatoes, ½ c margarine, cheese, onions, sour cream, soup and spices. Place in oiled 9x 13 inch casserole. Sprinkle corn flakes on top and pour the margarine on top. Bake uncovered in 350 ovens for 1 hour and 15 minutes.

Irene Williams

ENTREES

CHINESE *TUNO CASSEROLE

14 OZ CAN Chinese vegetables, drained

1 can mushroom soup

1 can *TUNO(Loma Linda)

¾ c celery, thinly sliced

1 t soy sauce

3 oz can Chinese noodles

Preheat oven to 350 degrees. Mix all ingredients except noodles in ungreased casserole dish. Sprinkle with noodles, bake uncovered until contents are bubbly and noodles golden brown about 40-45 minutes. Serve with rolls and salad.

Serves: 4

HASH BROWN POTATO CASSEROLE

1 (32oz) hash brown potatoes, frozen

½ c butter, melted · 8 oz cheese, shredded

1 c onions, chopped · 1 pt sour cream

1 can mushroom soup · salt & pepper

½ c corn flakes · ¼ c melted margarine

Defrost potatoes and mix ½ c margarine, cheese, sour cream, soup and spices. Put into a oiled 9x13 inch casserole. Sprinkle corn flakes on top and pour on margarine on top bake uncovered in 350 oven for 1 hour 15 minutes.

Irene Williams

GLUTEN STEAKS

4c. instant gluten flour · 1 c wheat flour

½ c minute tapioca · 4 T yeast flakes

3 T garlic powder · ¼ c soy sauce

3 ½ c cold water · 3 T chicken style seasonings

Mix dry ingredients well and add the liquid ingredients. Mix fast and knead. Shape into 2 rolls, wrap in plastic and freeze until almost solid. Slice to desired thickness then add to broth.

BROTH:

8 c. water · 1 onion, chopped

½ c soy sauce · 4 T yeast flakes

2 T oil · 3 T *McKay's chicken style broth mix

Put all ingredients in a pot and bring to a full boil. Drop gluten into pot and let boil for 20 minutes. Remove and store in a freezer container for future use.

FRIED GLUTEN

2 egg whites   2 T soy sauce
yeast flakes

Mix eggs and soy sauce in small bowl. Dip gluten steaks and cover with yeast flakes and fry until golden on both sides. Excellent served with favorite gravy.

Betty G. Perry

"CHICKEN" WITH TOMATOE SAUCE

2 13 OZ cans chicken style vegan-meat cut into bite size pieces
3-6 T oil   2 t salt
1 onion, thinly sliced
 5-6 tomatoes, mashed
4 stalks celery, diced
2 chili peppers, diced   (may substitute cayenne or hot sauce)

Fry chik vegan—meat in oil until golden brown. Remove *chiks and cook onions until golden. Return *chiks to pot and add remaining ingredients. Reduce heat and simmer for 15 minutes to blend flavors.

Serves: 8   Martha Bethea

CHICKEN GREEN BEAN ALFREDO

6 OZ dried fettuccine   4oz Alfredo sauce
2 cans green beans, drained
1 small can *Fri-chiks, sliced
Fresh basil

Cook pasta according to package, drain and return to sauce pan. Heat sauce, green beans and Chik in saucepan. Toss in pasta and sprinkle parmesan cheese. Transfer to serving dish and garnish with basil.

Martha Bethea

EGGPLANT PATTIES

1 eggplant, diced	½ c wheat germ
½ c walnuts, ground	½ c bread crumbs
½ c dry oatmeal	½ t salt
½ t. garlic powder	

Cook eggplant in salted water until soft, drain and mash. Add remaining ingredients and allow to stand to absorb moisture. Form into patties and brown in oil. Serve with brown gravy or tomato sauce.

Serves: 4   Rudene Morton

LOWFAT VEGETABLE LASAGNA

1 ½ c onions, diced	1 t. basil
3 cloves garlic, minced	½ t oregano
1 med eggplant, peeled and sliced	
½ t. fennel seeds	¼ c parsley, chopped
1 c zucchini, diced	2 c broccoli, chopped
9 lasagna noodles, cooked	
15 oz ricotta cheese	1 ½ c water, divided
4 c spaghetti sauce	
1 c nonfat mozzarella cheese	

Sauté' onions, garlic, eggplant and zucchini in skillet sprayed with *Pam. Add broccoli and 3 T of water and cover. Preheat oven to 350 degrees. To assemble lasagna, pour 1 c spaghetti sauce on the bottom of a 9x13 pan. Place 3 noodles on bottom and spread with ½ ricotta cheese, then with ½ vegetable mixture. Add another layer of sauce and 3 more noodles then the ricotta cheese, mozzarella cheese and 3 more noodles and cover with remaining sauce. Cover tightly and bake for 1 hour. Let sit for 10 minutes before serving.

SLOPPY JOES

1 can *Vegan-burger

1 can sloppy Joe sauce

Oil

Sauté' burger in oil until brown. Add sauce and continue to stir until bubbly. Serve on buns.

Betty Jordan

PINTO BEANS AND POTATOES

4 cups canned pinto beans	1 t. salt
2 lg. potatoes, chopped	1 onion, sliced
2 celery stalks, chopped	4 T.oil

Cook potatoes, add pinto beans, celery and salt. Cooke over low heat until tender. Fry onions in oil in a heavy stew pot. Using a slotted spoon add beans and potatoes to onion pot and serve well. Serve over rice.

Serves: 8

Martha Bethea

BAKED SLICED EGGPLANT

2 c bread crumbs	½ t. paprika
½ t. onion salt	½ t. salt
Soy mayo	eggplant, sliced ½ " thick

Mix bread crumbs and seasonings. Add enough water to mayo to make it easy for dipping the eggplant. Dip slices in the mayo and cover with bread crumbs. Bake on an oiled baking sheet until brown.

Serves:6

Rudene Morton

SAVORY RED BEANS

2 cans red kidney beans	2T olive oil
1 l. onion, chopped	6 c broth
2 celery ribs sliced	1 t. Thyme
1 green bell pepper, chopped	salt
2 cloves garlic, minced	2 bay leaves
1 t. crushed red pepper	1 t sea salt

Sauté' veggies in oil then add to beans and simmer for 30-40 minutes. Delicious when served over rice.

Irene Williams

PERFECT RICE

1 ½ long grain rice	2 ½ c broth
1 t. sea salt	2 t. oil

Sauté' uncooked rice in oil for 2-3 minutes, then add broth or water and cook for about 15 minutes.

Serves : 4   Martha Bethea

*CHICKEN LOAF

1 can *Chik, diced	2 c bread crumbs
1 t onion, chopped	2 T. oil
½ c milk	½ c peppers & celery
1 can cream of celery soup	

Sauté' vegetables in oil. Combine all ingredients and pour into an oiled loaf pan and bake for 45 minutes at 350 degrees. Excellent served with mushroom gravy.

Annie Flowers

ENTREES
PERFECT OAT PATTIES

8 c oats	1 onion, chopped
1 c walnuts, chopped	1 c sunflower seeds
1 c *Braggs Liquid Amino	1 T basil
1/3 nutritional yeast flakes	
2 T Italian seasoning	2 t oregano

Boil 8 cups water and 1 c *Braggs. Mix with other ingredients in large bowl and let sit for 20 minutes. Shape into patties using a 1/3 c scoop. Place on prepare baking sheet and bake at 350 degree oven for 25 minutes on one side and 20 minutes on other side. Let cool on a rack. These taste better the next day and freeze well.

Martha Bethea

*CHIK N BEAN CASSEROLE

1 CAN *Fri-chik	eggs, beaten
1 c bread crumbs	1 t. mustard
1 onion, chopped, 1 clove garlic	
1 t. Worcestershire sauce	
1 box frozen Italian beans, thawed	

Dip each *Fri.-chik into beaten eggs and then into bread crumbs and place in casserole and cook covered on high for 2 minutes. Remove *chiks from casserole and place the thawed beans in bottom of dish. Combine the other ingredients for the sauce. Place the chiks on top of the beans and then pour sauce over all and cook for 5-7 more minutes.

*"CHIK" CHOW MEIN

1 can *Fri-Chik, cut into 1.2 "cubes

2 c celery, thinly sliced

1 c onion thinly sliced

2 T cornstarch

¼ c water

1 can Chinese vegetables, drained

1 t brown sauce or molasses

2 T soy sauce

¼ t. ginger, ground

1 T. cornstarch

1 c chicken style broth

Stir Fri-Chik, celery, onion, 2 T cornstarchs and ¼ c water and microwave for 4 minutes. Add Chinese vegetables, brown sauce or molasses, 2 T soy sauce and ¼ t ginger.
Blend 1T cornstarch with ¼ c broths then add the rest of the broth; blend all in with the casserole and cook for 2-3 minutes. Serve with rice or noodles.

ENTREES
SAUCY GINGER CHIK

1can *Fri-chik	¼ t onion, garlic, ginger
powder	
2 eggs, beaten	2 T apple juice
¼ c Parmesan cheese	1 stick butter
2 c seasoned bread crumbs	

Combine bread crumbs and cheese. Mix eggs with apple juice. Season *fri-chik with spices and dip into egg mixture and then to bread crumbs. Place in microwaveable baking dish and pour butter all and bake for 12 minutes. Serve with favorite sauce.
Serves: 4

TOFU RIBS

2 lbs frozen tofu, thawed, squeezed dry and cut into rib-like strips
1 c barbeque sauce

Oil or spray a 9x12 pan. Place tofu strips leaving space between each strip. Bake for 10-15 minutes or until browned, turn over and brown opposite side. Remove from oven and pour thin layer of barbeque sauce on bottom of pan. Layer strip and sauce and make sure they are well covered. Let marinated overnight. Heat oven 375 degrees for 10-15 minutes.

Delicious served over rice, noodles or a sandwich.

Martha Bethea

*CHIK N DRESSING

1 corn bread, prepared   1 stick butter
½ c celery, peppers and onion, chopped
1 T. *Chicken –style seasoning
1 can *Fri Chik, sliced   1 can mushrooms
2 c. hot water   ½ t sage

Sauté' veggies, then add all ingredients together and place in baking dish. Arrange *Fri-Chiks on top, cover and bake for 45 minutes. Serve with gravy and cranberry sauce.

Betty G. Perry

POTATO PATTIES

2 lg. onions, diced   1 t. sage
1 c walnut pieces   2 c. bread crumbs
2 c potato with skins   2 eggs
Garlic salt   liquid smoke
1-2 t. soy sauce

Mix well and make into patties. Fry in oil. Excellent served with tomato sauce or gravy.

Pastor S. Perry

STIR-FRY VEG-CHOP

1 can *Choplets, slivered

1 onion, slivered	1 c. carrots, julienne
1 c peppers, julienne	2 c. celery, slivered
1 can mushrooms	1/3 c oil
Soy sauce	2 c cooked rice (add 1/4t turmeric
to cooking water)	

Stir fry all ingredients except rice until tender in oil until tender, season with soy sauce and serve over rice.

Annie Flowers

PECAN NUT PATTIES

1 ½ c cottage cheese	6 eggs, beaten
1 c pecans, ground	1 t. sage
Seasonings	favorite sauce
¼ c oil	1 c seasoned bread crumbs

Peppers, celery and onions chopped

Sauté' veggies in oil, then combine other ingredients except sauce. Form into balls and drop into hot oil until browned.

Place into covered baking dish and pour favorite sauce and place in oven for 5 minutes at 350 degrees.

Betty G. Perry

RED BEANS AND RICE

1 med. onion, chopped   2 cloves garlic

½ green and red peppers, chopped

4 c. vegetable stock   bay leaf

4 15oz cans tomatoes, chopped

1 t salt free Creole seasoning

½ t. cumin   ½ t thyme

Fresh ground pepper or hot sauce

2 cans red beans

Sauté' the vegetables in the oil. Pour the broth in large pot and add all ingredients and let simmer for 25 minutes. Serve with brown or white rice

Serves: 6-8   Martha Bethea

GLUTEN

Unbleached flour   seasonings

Water

1. Make flour into a dough ball. Put in large container and cover with water. Let sit at least 4 hours.

2. Rinse all starch out of dough for gluten. Water should be clear when starch is out.

3.Add seasonings to boiling water and place desired amount gluten in water to serve for chop lets or ground burger.

Morna Thompson

ENTREES

*CHIC AND NOODLES

1 lg. can *Fri-Chik	12 oz. noodles
2 can mushroom soup	1c celery, diced
1 c onions, diced	1 stick butter
1 can milk	

Boil noodles in salted water with 1 T. oil and drain. Cut *Fri-Chik into small pieces and set aside. Sauté' celery and onions in oil. Put all ingredients into large baking dish and mix well. Bake at 350 degree oven for 30 minutes.

Morna Thompson

*SWISS STEAK PARMESEAN

1 can *Swiss Steaks

1 onion sliced   ¼ c olive oil

1 c *Kellogg's Bread Crumbs

1 jar spaghetti sauce

1 c mozzarella cheese, shredded

Dredge steaks in bread crumbs, and brown both sides in olive oil. Pour half of spaghetti sauce in large baking dish and arrange steaks in one layer. Sauté' onion, then place onions and cheese on each steak and add the remainder spaghetti sauce. Bake at 350 degrees for 30 minutes or until bubbly.

Serves: 8   Betty G. Perry

TAMALE PIE

2 c *Crumbles

2 c corn chips, crumbled   ¼ c olive oil

1 pkg. taco seasoning mix   1 c salsa

½ c black olives, sliced   1 c corn

1 c cheese, shredded

Combine all ingredients, stir well. Place in large oiled baking dish and bake at 350 degrees for 35 minutes.

Serve: 8

*CHICK-RAGUT

1 Lg. Can *Fri-Chik   1 onion, sliced

1 c mozzarella cheese   spaghetti sauce

¼ c olive oil   1 c bread crumbs

Dredge each chik in bread crumbs and fry until brown on both sides. Sauté' onion. Pour spaghetti sauce in large baking dish, then add the chiks, followed by a layer of onion and cheese. Put remaining sauce over chiks and bake at 350 degrees for 30 minutes.

Serves: 8   Patricia Davis

WINTER SQUASH CASSEROLE

2 c mashed squash	4 *breakfast strips
1 onion, chopped	¾ c cheddar , shredded
Seasoning	cayenne pepper
½ c bread crumbs	¼ c oil

Oil a small baking dish. Brown the breakfast strips. Sauté' onions in oil Place squash in bowl with all ingredients except bread crumbs, then pour into baking dish and top with bread crumbs. Place in oven for 30 minutes or until brown.

Serves: 4

SPAGHETTI

1 CAN *Redi-burger	spaghetti sauce
1 lb spaghetti, cooked	1/3 c olive oil
Parmesan cheese	3 cloves garlic
1c onion, celery and peppers, minced	

Sauté' veggies in oil, then brown *Redi burger in same skillet. Combine all ingredients well and serve.

Annie Flowers

Stop! Do not pour the liquids from can goods down the sink. Instead pour into a designated ice tray until it is full. Then empty the frozen ice tray juices into a plastic bag to store in the freezer. When you are ready for broth or gravy additions you will have it, just drop a few "veggie flavor cubes". Have 2 designated trays one for the veggies and one for fruits. Fruit flavor cubes are tasty when added to smoothies, punch or desserts.

LENTIL ROAST

2 c lentils, cooked	¼ t salt
1c potatoes, diced, cooked	1 T *Vegex
4 T butter	1 can mushrooms
2 T flour	2c milk

Sauté' onions, add *vegex, flour then milk and cook a few minutes. Combine all ingredients and pour into a greased baking dish. Bake at 350 degrees for 20 minutes. Serve with a tossed salad.

Annie Flowers

PINEAPPLE-*WHAM ENTRÉE

1 pkg. *Wham slices	2 T corn starch
½ c brown sugar	cloves
¼ c raisins	1 stick butter
Pineapple chunks	1 ½ c pineapple juice

Melt butter in flat casserole and place wham slices individually with pineapple rings or chunks. In small sauce pan combine cloves, sugar, pineapple juice and cornstarch and heat to thicken. Pour over the wham pineapple slices and bake in oven for 20 minutes. Garnish with maraschino cherries.

Serves: 4-6 Martha Bethea

ENTREES
COTTAGE CHEESE LOAF

1 qt. cottage cheese	1 pkg. onion soup mix
1 c walnuts, chopped	3 eggs
1 c bread crumbs	½ c bread crumbs
1 celery stalk, diced ½ c peppers, diced	
¼ c oil	1 c broth

Combine all ingredients and bake in oiled casserole at 350 degrees for 1 hour.

Serves: 8-10   Annie Flowers

ORIENTAL RICE

3 c cooked rice	3 scrambled eggs
1 can bean sprouts	1 can mushrooms
¼ c oil	soy sauce
1 can *Fri chiks, diced	
1 c chopped celery, green onion, peppers	

Sauté' veggies until tender. Combine all ingredients in skillet mixing well. Transfer to serving dish.

Serves: 8   Betty G. Perry

VEGE –STROGANOFF

1 lg. can *Vegan-meat	3 T. oil
1 pkg. onion soup mix	1 c sour cream
1 can mushrooms	2 T flour
2/3 c water	1 8oz noodles, cooked

Cut vegan-meat in strips and brown in oil. Add mushrooms and onion soup mix and flour, heat to boiling and add sour cream. Cook until sauce thickens. Serve over hot noodles or rice

Annie Flowers

MUSHROOM NUT ROAST

3 cans mushroom	1 c nuts, chopped
1 stick butter	1 c cheese, grated
1 onion, chopped	4 eggs, beaten
1/4c steak sauce	1 pkg. dressing mix

Mix all ingredients well and pour into an oiled casserole. Bake at 350 degrees for 30 minutes. Blend ¼ c steak sauce with ¼ c water and pour over the top and bake for 30 minutes more. Serve with mushroom sauce.

MUSHROOM SAUCE

1 can mushroom soup

1 pint sour cream

1 can mushrooms

Mix all ingredients and simmer for 10 minutes.

Serves: 8-10

Betty G. Perry

ENTREES
CHOPLETS QUICK ENTRÉE

1 can *chop lets	½ c oil
2 onions	1 egg
1 c bread crumbs	2 T flour
1 can cream soup	

Drain *Choplets and reserve liquid. Dip into beaten egg and then into bread crumbs. Brown in skillet and remove to a flat casserole dish. Sauté' onions in oil and place over the *chop lets. In skillet brown flour, add liquid and cream soup and water as necessary for desired consistency. Pour sauce over onions and chop-lets. Cover with bread crumbs and bake at 350 degrees oven for 30 minutes.

Serves: 6-8   Irene Williams

*CHIK TETRAZZINI

4 oz thins spaghetti, broken and cooked

1 c milk	1 onion, diced
1 c shredded cheese	1 cup *chik, diced
¼ c pimento, chopped	½ c milk
1 can mushroom soup	¼ c pepper, diced
½ c sour cream	

Sauté' peppers and onions, then combine all ingredients except ½ of the cheese to sprinkle on top. Place in an oiled casserole dish and bake at 400 degrees for 30 minutes.

Irene Williams

CHOP SUEY

1 c thinly sliced celery and leaves

1 c sliced onions & peppers

1 c broth   1 T cornstarch

2 c slivered *Fri-Chiks

1 can chop suey vegetables or bean sprouts, drained

1 can water chestnuts, sliced and drained

2 T soy sauce   1 c toasted almonds

Hot cooked rice   4 T oil

Sauté' vegetables in oil. Add broth and cornstarch, cooking until thickened. Add all ingredients except rice. Heat well, serve over rice or noodles.

Irene Williams

ENTREES

VEGEBURGER LOAF

1 can *vegan-burger	1 onion, minced
1 c dry breadcrumbs	1 pepper, minced
2 stalks celery, diced	2 eggs
½ c pecans, chopped	¼ t thyme, sage
1-2 c cream soup	2 cloves garlic,
¼ c oil	minced

Sauté' veggies, then combine all ingredients and place in an oiled pan. Bake at 350 degrees for 1 hour. Serve with favorite gravy.

Serves: 8-10   Irene Williams

STUFFED BELL PEPPERS

8 bell peppers, cored

Parmesan cheese, grated

Spaghetti sauce

Parboil peppers for 5 minutes. When cool stuff with vegan-burger recipe above. Spread layer of spaghetti sauce in casserole dish, and then place stuffed peppers, pouring spaghetti sauce and parmesan cheese over the top. Bake in 350 degree oven for 1 hour.

Serves: 8   Betty G. Perry

FROSTED MEAT LOAF DINNER

2 c bread crumbs	½ c onions, chopped
Salt & Pepper	½ c milk
1 pkg. *Crumbles	2 eggs, beaten
4 c mashed potatoes	paprika
1 1/c cheese, shredded	
1 pkg. frozen mixed vegetables, cooked	

Mix all ingredients together, except the last 4. Shape and form into a ring loaf. Bake in microwave high for 5 minutes. Remove loaf inverting to a platter. Frost loaf ring with mashed potatoes, sprinkle cheese on top, return to oven to melt cheese Sprinkle top with paprika and fill center with mixed vegetables.

Serves: 4   Irene Williams

ONION CHEESE PIE

2 prepared pie crusts	2 c cheese, shred.
1 can mushroom soup	2c onions, diced
Salt and pepper	½ stick butter
1 T flour	

In bottom pie crust sprinkle the flour, then layer onions, salt and pepper, cheese, butter and mushroom soup. Place top crust on and seal. Bake in 350 degree oven for 35-40 minutes until brown.

Serves: 8   Betty G. Perry

ENTREES

Walnut Burgers

4 c walnuts, ground	1 c wheat flour
2 c oatmeal	1-2 c salsa
Peppers, celery and onion, diced	
1 jalapeño, chopped	3T mustard
½ c mayo	1 egg
1/3 c Worchester sauce	¼ c oil

Combine all ingredients and make into patties and fry or place in oiled loaf pan and bake at 350 degrees for 45 minutes.

Serve: 30   Irene Williams

Mexican "Beef" and Rice

1 pkg. *Crumbles	salt & pepper
8 green onions, sliced	1 can tomato sauce
1 c water	¼ c olives, sliced
1 T chili powder	1 ½ c *Minute rice
Hot peppers	tortilla chips

Combine all ingredients except tortilla chips in a microwave dish, cover and cook on high for 5 minutes, stir and cook 5 minutes more. Let stand for 5 minutes; fluff with fork. Serve with tortilla chips.

Serves: 8   Irene Williams

TURKEY STYLE MEATBALLS

1 pkg. *Turkey –style slices, ground	
1 onion, diced	½ c bread crumbs
1 ½ T cold water	1 egg
Seasonings	½ t *Mrs. Dash
2 T cooking oil	1pkg brown gravy mix

In bowl combine all ingredients except oil and gravy mix. Shape mixture into meat balls. In hot skillet with oil, brown the meat balls. In large saucepan mix gravy mix according to instructions. Add meatballs and simmer for 1 hour. Serve with cooked noodles or rice.

TURKEY BAKE

1 BOX *Turkey style slices, ground

2 cans tomatoes   1 cream celery soup

1 can mushroom soup   2 T. butter

1 c *Minute Rice, uncooked

1 c cheddar, grated

2 c tortilla chips, crushed

Mix together all ingredients except tortilla chips and cheddar cheese. Spread butter in bottom of 13x9 inch pan and cover with 1 c crush chips. Pour in ground turkey mixture, sprinkle grated cheese on top and cover with 1 c crushed chips. Bake at 350 degrees for 45 minutes to an hour.

Betty G. Perry

ENTREES

CORN FLAKE ROAST

5 C *Kellogg's Corn Flakes   2 eggs

2 c. milk   ¼ c oil

1 pkg. onion soup mix   1 onion, diced

5 ribs celery, chopped   1 T* McKay's

Chik seasoning

Put all ingredients in a large bowl and toss. Pour milk over all and mix well Cook in a greased casserole 8x8 dish for 30 minutes at 350 degrees. Add your favorite gravy over casserole before serving or use plain.

Serves: 6-8   Bobbie Drummond

*SWISS STEAK CASSEROLE

1 small can *Swiss steak

½ onion, chopped

1 t. Italian seasoning

1 c water

can mushroom

1 t. garlic powder

1 pkg. brown gravy

Place *Swiss steak in oiled casserole dish. Mix all other ingredients together. Cover *Swiss steak with mixture. Bake for 40 minutes at 350 degrees.

Serves: 4-6   Jessie White

CHICKEN GREEN BEAN ALFREDO

8 oz fettuccine, cooked

1 ½ c *Alfredo sauce

2 cans green beans, drained

1 ½ c *vegan chi ken strips

3 T Parmesan cheese

onion, diced

¼ t basil

Sauté' green beans, onions and vegan strips and basil for 3-5 minutes. Add past. Serve on platter with cheese sprinkled on top.

Serves: 4-6   Martha Bethea

GERMAN GREENBEANS AND TOMATOES

1 lb fresh green beans,

green onion, chopped

3 tomatoes, chopped 1t.*McCormick

seasoning

½ c sour cream

3 T. wine vinegar

Cook green beans, drain and keep warm. Sprinkle chopped onions on top. In bowl, mix together sour cream.

Martha Bethea

ENTREES
BARBEQUE CHICKS

1 roll *Worthington Chicks

Olive oil

Barbeque sauce

Cut chicks in bite sized pieces then brush with oil and brown in oven. Arrange in baking pan and pour barbeque sauce over and return to oven until bubbly.

BBQ MEATBALLS

1 bag *CRUMBLES	1 onion, chopped
½ red & green bell peppers	
1 c cheese, shredded	1 c bread crumbs
½ c bread crumbs	½ c pecan meals
2 cloves garlic, minced	1/4 c olive oil
Sage, thyme, salt & pepper	

Sauté' veggies in oil then combine all ingredients in a medium mixing bowl. Shape into meatballs and place on a sprayed baking sheet. Place in 375 degree oven for 20 minutes. Pour *BBQ sauce over the meatballs and return to oven for 5-7 minutes.

Serves: 8   Betty G. Perry

MILLETT PATTIES

1 c. cooked millet	3 cloves garlic, minced
2 T flour	1 onion, chopped
¼ c walnuts, chopped	1 lb tofu, crumbled
½ c bread crumbs	1 t. basil
2 t nutritional yeast	4 t *McKay's Chick

Oregano, sage, thyme, salt & pepper

2 T olive oil

Combine all ingredients well and shape into patties, placing into an oiled baking sheet. Bake at 350 degrees oven until brown and turn once. Serve with favorite gravy.

FISH—CHICK PATTIES

1 roll frozen *vegan Tuno	olive oil
1 can vegan *Fri-Chick, shredded	
1 lb tofu, crumbled	onion, chopped
*McKay's Chick to taste	½ c bread crumbs

Sauté' onion in olive oil. Combine all ingredients and form into patties and place on sprayed baking sheet. Bake at 400 degrees until browned turning once.

Serves: 10   Irene Williams

ENTREES
WALNUT BALLS

1 c ground raw potatoes	2 t. flour
1 c wheat flour	lg. onion, chopped
1 c. ground walnuts	½ t sage
Salt & pepper	¼ c oil

Mix all ingredients thoroughly and form into balls. Put in baking dish and pour favorite gravy over them. Bake at 375 degrees for 20-30 minutes.

Serves: 4-6   Florine Tyler

CHICKEN ROAST

2 c bread crumbs	1 ½ c water
1 c onion, chopped	1 celery, chopped
3 T oil	2 *T McKay's Chick
4 ½ c *chick soy meat, ground	
2 T. soy flour	
½ t. salt	
1 c milk	

Mix bread crumbs in water. Sauté' onions and celery in oil and add to bread crumbs. Mix in all remaining ingredients. Pour into greased casserole dish. Bake for 1 hour at 350 degrees.

Serves: 6-8   Bobbie Drummond

OATNUT BURGER

2 c. dry oatmeal   1c. pecan meal

1 ½ t Italian seasoning   salt & pepper

Sage

1 can evap. Milk or soy milk

Combine above ingredients and let stand for 15-20 minutes.

In a skillet, sauté':

1 chopped onion,

1 c. chopped celery,

1 bell pepper

In 2 T oil then add to first mixture. Form into small patties. Fry over medium heat until brown on both sides. Place in baking dish. Dilute a can of cream of mushroom soup with desired thickness and pour over patties. You may opt to use your favorite gravy or tomato sauce instead of mushroom soup.

Bake for 15 minutes more at 375 degrees.

Serve 4-6   Bobbie Drummond

Healthy Hint:

When boiling rice or potatoes the addition of "veggie flavor cubes"(broth) as a portion of the liquid is nice.

ENTREES

BASIC MACARONI AND CHEESE

3 T liquid butter buds   1 ½ T flour

½ t. salt & pepper   2 c milk

c elbow or shell macaroni, cooked

1 T onion, grated

c cheddar cheese, shredded

½ c seasoned bread crumbs

Prepare a white sauce in a pan by combining milk, flour, butter buds, salt & pepper. Stir with wire whisk until thickened, set aside. Place half of cooked macaroni in bottom of sprayed casserole dish, then sprinkle half of onions and cheese, then add the other half of macaroni sprinkle the remaining cheese over it. Pour the sauce over and sprinkle with bread crumbs. Cover and bake for 30 minutes then uncover and bake for 10 minutes longer.

Serves: 8   Naomi Thompson

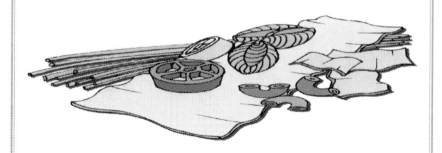

TAMALE PIE

Cornmeal Mush:

1 lg. bag corn chips, crushed

Filling:

2 T. oil	2 c *Crumbles
Salt & pepper	1 can corn
1 c black olives, sliced	1 can tomato sauce

1 onion, bell pepper 1 clove garlic, chopped

½ t cumin 1 T soy sauce

1 pkg. taco seasoning

½ c cheddar, shredded

Sauté' veggies then mix all filling ingredients. Layer bottom of casserole with crushed corn chips. Then pour in the filling

Garnish with black olives and cheddar cheese. Bake at 350 degrees for 1 hour.

Serves: 8-10 Irene Williams

ENTREES
QUICK & EASY MEATBALLS

1 pkg. *Crumbles	1 c cheese, shredded
1 c bread crumbs	2 eggs
1 can mushroom soup	1 onion, diced
½ c salsa sauce	dash thyme
Dash taco seasoning	1 pkg. broth
¼ c oil	

Combine all ingredients well, make into small melon size balls. Place onto an oil baking sheet and bake 350 degree oven for 25 minutes. Serve with your favorite sauce or gravy.

Yield: 2 dozen   Betty G. Perry

MOM'S MACARONI & CHEESE

1 ½ c macaroni, cooked	2T butter
1 small onion, chopped	¼ c flour
Salt & pepper	1 ¾ c milk
6 oz cheese, cubed	

Heat oven to 375 degrees. In saucepan melt butter and sauté' onions, adding salt and pepper. Mix flour and milk until smooth, stir into onion mixture. Heat to boiling, stirring constantly for 1 minute. Remove from heat and stir in cheese until melted. Combine the cheese mixture with macaroni dish and bake for 30 minutes, or until lightly browned.

Serves: 5   Naomi Thompson

IRENE'S POTATO MEAL

2 ½ lbs white potatoes, cubed

Bell peppers, celery, jalapenos, onion, garlic, diced

1 c mayo	4 T mustard
Lemon or lime juice	1c salsa-cheese
Parsley flakes	salt & pepper

Stir well and enjoy

Serves: 10-12   Irene Williams

VEGETABLE JUMBO SHELLS

12 jumbo pasta shells, cooked

1 carrot, chopped	1 can broth
1 potato, cubed	1 zucchini, cubed
1/2 c broccoli, chopped	1 T basil

2 t parmesan cheese, grated

2 T bread crumbs

Preheat oven to 400 degrees. Heat broth to boiling in saucepan. Stir in carrot and potato cooking 2-4 minutes then stir in zucchini and broccoli, cooking for 1 minute. Add I t. of the cheese and 1 t of the bread crumbs to the vegetables. Fill cooked shells with vegetable mixture and place in a square baking dish, fill side up. Add reserved broth to pan. Mix remaining cheese and bread crumbs and sprinkle over shells. Bake uncovered 10-12 minutes or until golden. To serve spoon broth from dish over shells.

Serve: 5-6   Irene Williams

ENTREES

HARVEST NUT ROAST

2 ½ celery, chopped

3 T water

¾ c walnuts, chopped

1 ½ t. salt

2 ½ c soymilk

½ t. sage

3 onions, chopped

2 T oil

¾ c pecan meal

3 c bread crumbs

1 ¼ t. basil

Sauté' vegetables in water and oil, then combine with remaining ingredients. Place in oiled loaf pan and bake for 1 ½ hrs at 350 degrees. After 45 minutes cover top with foil. Serve with gravy.

Serves: 8   Rudene Morton

*SWISS STEAK CASSEROLE

1 small can *Swiss steak

½ onion, sliced

1 t. Italian seasoning

1 prepared brown gravy

1 t. garlic powder

1 can mushrooms

1 c water

Combine all ingredients and bake at 350 degree oven for 40 minutes.

Serves: 4   Mary Alford

*CHIK SALAD

1 can *Fri-chik

Celery, diced

Pimientos

onion, diced

pickles, diced

mayo

Grate or mash *Chik, add all ingredients according to taste.

Mary Alford

CHICKEN ROAST

2 c bread crumbs

1 c onion, chopped

1 c. celery, chopped

4 c ground *Fri-chik

1 c milk

2 c broth

3 T oil

2 T. soy flour

½ t salt

2 t *McKay's Chik

Sauté' all vegetables in oil. Mix with all ingredients and pour into a greased casserole dish. Bake for 1 hour at 350 degrees.

Serves: 4   Bobbie Drummond

HINT!

Pour all leftover vegetable juices into a freezer container. When full add tomato juice and seasoning to create a "free soup".

ENTREES

VEGETARIAN LASAGNA

1 lb box lasagna noodles, cooked

6 c marinara sauce

24 oz cottage cheese

32 oz mozzarella cheese, shredded

½ c basil, oregano or thyme

2 eggplants, cut circular slices

6-8 zucchini, cut lengthwise

5 Portobello mushroom, thinly sliced

2 red onions, thinly sliced

4 T olive oil

4 cloves garlic, minced

¾ c onions, chopped

2 28 oz cans diced tomatoes

1/3 c basil, chopped

Sauté' or oven roast all vegetables until cooked through and set aside. To the sauce add herbs, chopped onion and garlic. Pour some sauce on the bottom of a 9x12 baking dish and place a layer of noodles, followed by a layer of vegetables and cheese. Keep layering for 3 layers. Top with noodles and sauce. Bake at 350 degrees for 30-40 minutes.

Serves: 10-12   Martha Bethea

*TUNO BURGERS

1 CAN *TUNO	cayenne, dash
3-4 T onion, chopped	soy sauce, dash
1 stalk celery, chopped	salt & pepper
½ c bread crumbs	4 T. oil

Sauté' the vegetables. Combine all ingredients and make into 4 separate patties. Brown on both sides in a skillet, serve as a sandwich or as an entrée with your favorite sauce.

Serves: 4

A slice of cheese would make a nice Tuno melt

GLAZED * TUNO BURGERS

*Tuno Burgers:

1 can* tuno	salt and pepper
Cayenne, dash	olive oil
Burger buns	

Mustard Glaze:

2 t minced garlic	2t Dijon mustard
1/3 c honey	1/3 c teriyaki sauce
½ t vinegar	

Combine burger ingredients into 4 patties and brown both sides in a skillet. Turn them then add the combines ingredients for the glaze. Allow to set for a few minutes and serve.

ENTREES

GLAZED *TUNO

1 c pineapple juice	¼ c vinegar
3 T soy sauce	3 T soy sauce
3 t. brown sugar	3 T lime juice
1 can* Tuno	

Mix first five ingredients together in sauce pan and heat for 3-5 minutes. Divide the *tuno mixture into 2-4 patties. Brown in a skillet then pour the pineapple mixture over.

VEGETABLES
SPINACH NOODLE CASSEROLE

1lb noodles, cooked	6 T butter
2 boxes spinach, cooked	salt &pepper
1 pt sour cream	
2 can mushroom soup	
½ onion, chopped	

Sauté' mushrooms and onions in butter. Butter a large casserole dish. Mix together all ingredients, place in casserole, bake at 350 degrees for 30 minutes or until bubbly.

Serves: 6

BROCCOLI CASSEROLE

¼ c onion, chopped	6 T butter
½ c water	2 T flour
8 oz cheese spread	3 eggs
½ c bread crumbs	
2 pkg. frozen chopped broccoli	

Sauté' onion in butter, stir in flour and add water. Cook over low heat, stirring until it thickens. Blend in cheese, combine sauce and broccoli. Add eggs, mix gently, turn into a 2 qt casserole and cover with crumbs and remaining butter. Bake for 30 minutes.

Serves: 8   Betty G. Perry

And broccoli sprouts may help protect stomachs in yet another way: by ramping up protective enzymes in stomach cells that help defend against damage. (Add an olive-oil-based dressing to your salad for even more *H. pylori* protection." So eat broccoli, for your stomach's sake and for better health. *(Source: Cancer Prevention Research 2009 Apr; 2(4):353-360.)*

YELLOW SQUASH CASSEROLE

2 lbs yellow squash, cooked, mashed

1 lg. onion, chopped	1c sour cream
1 can mushroom soup	salt & pepper
1 stick butter	8oz pkg. bread crumbs

Sauté' onion in half of butter; add soup, sour cream, salt and pepper. Melt remainder of butter and add to the bread crumbs. Put half of crumbs on bottom of casserole then put all of the squash followed by topping of crumbs. Bake at 350 degrees for 1 hour.

Serves: 8   Naomi Thompson

TURNIP CASSEROLE

1 ½ lbs turnips, thinly sliced and cooked

2 T butter	I onion thinly sliced
2/3c celery, bell pepper, chopped	
2 t flour	1 c milk
½ c cheese, grated	salt and pepper
3 T bread crumbs	

Sauté 'onion and celery in butter; sprinkle with flour and cook for 1 minute. Add milk and stir until thickened, stir in cheese, salt and pepper. Combine cheese sauce with turnips then place in baking dish and top with crumbs. Brown under broiler.

Serves: 4   Mary Alford

VEGETABLES
HARVEST VEGETABLE RICE

1 T butter	1 c onion, sliced
1 c mushrooms, sliced	
1 ½ c broth	1 ½ c instant brown rice
1 c sweet potatoes, shredded	
1 c broccoli florets	salt & pepper
¼ c cheese, shredded	

Melt butter in a saucepan, add onions and mushrooms and cook for 2 minutes. Add broth, rice, sweet potatoes, broccoli, salt and pepper. Bring to a boil and simmer for 10 minutes. Place mixture into a 2 qt. casserole dish and sprinkle with cheese, broil until cheese melts.

Serves: 4

ONION PIE

2 medium onions, thinly sliced

3 T butter	½ c milk
1 egg	½ c cheese, grated
½ c saltine crackers, crushed	

Preheat oven to 325 degrees and prepare a 7 inch pie plate with spray. Sauté' onions until transparent in 1 t butter then spread in prepared pie plate. Whisk egg and cheese and milk then pour over onions. Toast the cracker crumbs with butter in the skillet then sprinkle over the mixture. Bake 5-10 minutes or just until set.

Serves: 2   Betty G. Perry

VEGETABLE, BEAN RICE SALAD

1 c rice	1 ½ eggplant, cubed
1 can navy beans, rinsed	
3 tomatoes , diced	1/4c olives, chopped
1/3 c fresh basil, chopped	
1 sm. Zucchini, sliced	

DRESSING:

6 T chicken style broth	
2 t vinegar	
1 t. mustard,	1 clove garlic, minced

Prepare rice according to directions. During last 10 minutes of cooking add eggplant. Place rice mixture in a large bowl and let cool slightly. Add beans, tomatoes, zucchini, basil and olives, mix well.

Combine dressing ingredients in blender bowl and beat on high for 1 minute. Pour over rice mixture and toss.

Serves: 4

Healthy Hint:

In some entrees that call for broth, flavor cubes and broth are a wonderful combination.

VEGETABLES/ SIDES
CREAMED CABBAGE

1 med head cabbage	½ c cream
1 oz butter	seasonings
1 c water	

Slice cabbage as for slaw. Cook in 1 c water until tender, drain. Add cream and seasonings.

ZUCCHINI QUICHE

1 c corn muffin mix	3c zucchini
1 med onion, chopped	4 eggs, beaten
½ c parmesan cheese	1/3 c olive oil
Seasoning	1 c cream

Mix all together and pour into a oiled pan or pie plate and bake at 350 degrees for 45 minutes.

SAUCY ASPARAGUS

2 cans asparagus, drained	½ stick butter
1 can mushroom soup	mushrooms
4 oz cheese slices	1 ¼ c bread crumbs

Oil a long flat casserole dish and place asparagus on bottom. Add mushroom soup and mushroom pieces, cover with cheese slices. Put bread crumbs over cheese and thinly sliced butter on top. Bake 25 minutes in 350 degree oven or until bubbly.

Serves: 6

GERMAN GREEN BEANS

1 lb. Fresh green beans   ½ c. sour cream

1 bunch green onions, chopped

3 T. vinegar   3 tomatoes, chopped

1 t. *McCormick seasoning

Cook green beans, drain and keep warm, add vinegar and seasonings. Stir tomatoes and sour cream into beans and serve.

Serves: 4-6   Ethel Bell

SAVORY SUCCOTASH

1 can french style green beans, drained

1 can whole kernel corn, drained

½ c mayo   ½ c cheese, shredded

½c pepper, 1/2c celery, 2T. onions, chopped

1 c bread crumbs   2 T. butter, melted

Combine crumbs and butter. Combine remainder of ingredients and place in casserole 9x9. Sprinkle crumbs mixture on top. Bake in 350 degree oven or until crumbs are toasted.

Serves: 6   Betty Perry

VEGETABLES/SIDES
CORN PUDDING

1 egg   salt and pepper

1 t. sugar   1 T flour

1/3 c milk   1 can cream style corn

Preheat oven to 340 degrees. Oil a small baking dish. In a small bowl whisk egg, then add salt, pepper, sugar flour and milk. When smooth whisk in corn. Pour into prepared dish and bake until set firm when dish is giggled, about 35-40 minutes.

Serve: 2

THOUSAND ISLAND SALAD
DRESSING:

¼ c mayo

1 ½ T ketchup

1 ½ t pickle relish

½ green onion, chopped

SALAD:

Lettuce

3 hard cooked eggs

6 slices *Wham

Prepare dressing; combine all ingredients and mix well.

Cover 2 plates with chunks and leaves of lettuce. Top with *Wham and slices of eggs; spoon on dressing.

Serves: 2

GLAZED PARSNIPS

½ lb parsnips

1 T butter

2 T brown sugar

salt and pepper

Pinch nutmeg

1 T whipping cream

Half fill a medium saucepan with water; add salt, bring to boiling. Meanwhile prepare and trim parsnips. Cut in half lengthwise in uniform pieces. Drop into boiling water, cover cook for 5 minutes. Drain, rinse under cold water to stop the cooking, drain well. Melt butter in a shallow baking dish, add parsnips, and toss to coat with butter. Sprinkle on brown sugar, salt and pepper and nutmeg. Dribble on cream. Bake at 350 degrees about 20 minutes, stirring once to baste.

Serves: 2

VEGETABLES/SIDES
TWICE BAKED POTATOES

6 baking potatoes	salt and pepper
3 T butter	3 oz. cream cheese
1 2gg, beaten	1/3c cream

Bake potatoes for 1 hour at 450 degrees. Scoop out potato from skin and mash. In separate bowl combine the remaining ingredients and beat well. Fill the potato skins with this mixture and bake for 25 minutes at 400 degrees.

Serves: 6   Mary Alford

COMPANY MASHED POTATOES

4 c. hot, seasoned mashed potatoes

1 c. sour cream	1/3 c chopped onions
4 oz cheese, shredded	½ t. season salt

Combine all ingredients, except seasoned salt in greased casserole. Sprinkle with seasoned salt. Bake at 350 degrees for 25 minutes.

Naomi Thompson

BRAISED POTATOES

4 med. potatoes, quartered	3 T oil
1 T chicken style broth	
1 c boiling water	

Fry potatoes until browned. Dissolve the broth in boiling water and pour over potatoes. Cook covered for 10-15 minutes.

Pastor S. Perry

SOUR CREAM SCALLOPED POTATOES

½ c chopped onion   2T butter, melted
1 c. sour cream   2 eggs, beaten
Salt and pepper   1 c cheese, shredded
4 c potatoes, cooked and sliced

Sauté' onions in butter; combine with sour cream, eggs, salt and pepper. Place potatoes in buttered 1 qt. casserole and pour sour cream sauce over top. Then sprinkle with cheese. Bake 20-25 minutes at 350 degrees.
Serves: 6

CREAMED POTATOES

6 large potatoes, parboiled
½ lb butter, melted   salt and pepper
½ c heavy cream   ¾c. cheese, shredded

Let potatoes cool, break up into pieces coarsely, but do not mash. Place into a casserole. Add butter, salt and pepper and pour over potatoes then pour heavy cream and let stand for 10 minutes, then sprinkle with cheese. Bake 20 minutes in a 200 degree oven or until cheese is melted.
Serve: 6   Pastor S. Perry

Creamed Carrots

Bunch of carrots, scraped
Broth
½ c milk
½ stick butter

Boil carrots in broth until fork tender, remove and place in blender adding milk and butter then whiz it until smooth, add seasonings, mix again and serve as a side dish.
                    Betty Perry

VEGETABLES/SIDES
EGGPLANT CASSEROLE

2 eggplants, cubed and cooked

1 c breadcrumbs   1c cheese, shredded

Onion, peppers, celery, chopped

2 cloves garlic, minced

1 stick butter

2 T parsley, thyme, oregano

2 eggs, beaten

1 c *French's Onion toppers, crumbled

Combine all ingredients and place in an oiled casserole dish. Sprinkle onion toppers over the top. Bake at 350 degrees for 30 minutes.

Serves: 5-6

SAUSAGE CORNBREAD

1 cornbread mix   1 c buttermilk

1 pkg., *Breakfast patties

1 onion, chopped   ¼ c oil

1 egg

Sauté' onion and crumbles patties then combine all in a 400 degree oven for 25-30 minutes or browned. Enjoy.

For variation 1 cup of chopped broccoli and ½ c shredded cheeses can be used.

Serves: 8   Betty G. Perry

BETTY'S BURRITO

1 c rice, cooked	1 c *Crumbles
3 cloves garlic, crushed	2 c. salsa
Chili powder, sage, thyme	1/3 c oil
1 c cheese, shredded	1 can olives, sliced
1t crushed red peppers	seasonings
Corn tortillas	

Sauté' *crumbles then combine all ingredients except tortillas. Heat tortillas briefly in microwave and lay them open. Place 1-2 T of rice mixture in center of each tortilla and then roll it closed, placing the edges down in an oiled casserole dish. Continue until all mixture is used. Pour salsa' sauce overall and add shredded cheese on each and bake at 350 degrees for 10-15 minutes.

Serves: 10   Betty Perry

STUFFED TOMATOES

6 red tomatoes, inside removed

1 pkg. spinach	1 jar artichokes
1 c shredded cheese	¼ c. oil
2 cloves garlic, minced	½ c breadcrumbs
onions, peppers, chopped	

Combine all ingredients well. Using a tablespoon fill the tomatoes with the mixture and place on a oiled baking dish. Bake for25 minutes. Then place a bit of cheese on top for 5 minutes more.

Serves: 6

So include tomatoes and tomato sauces in your diet for better health. (Source: *International Journal of Cancer* April 15, 2009)

VEGETABLE/SIDE
SCALLOPED CHEESE POTATOES

¼ c butter	3 T. flour
2 t. dried chives and green onion	
Salt and pepper	
½ t dry mustard	1 ¾ c milk
4 med potatoes, sliced	
1 c. grated cheese	

Microwave butter in 2 qt. casserole for 45 seconds. Stir in flour, chives, salt and pepper, mustard. Blend in milk. Microwave on high for 6-7 minutes, or until thickened. Mix in potatoes and cheese, cover. Microwave on high for 15-20 minutes until potatoes are done. Stirring 2-3 times.

TACO MAIN DISH

1 bag *crumbles	1 onion, diced
¼ c oil	1 can kidney beans
Taco seasoning mix	1 can olives
1 can whole kernel corn	
1 can tomato sauce	
1 corn chips, crushed	

Brown *crumbles in microwave for 2 minutes. Add remaining ingredients and heat through, cover with grated cheese and heat until cheese melts.

Serves: 4

CHEESY ASPARAGUS

2 cans asparagus, drained   salt and pepper

2 hard boiled eggs, sliced

5 crackers, crushed

1 can cheddar soup

1 can mushrooms, drained

2 oz slivered almonds

½ c cheese, shredded   paprika

Place half of asparagus in a 2 qt. casserole. Sprinkle with ½ seasonings, top with ½ egg slices, mushrooms, almonds and crackers and ½ of soup, repeat layers. Microwave for 2 minutes or until cheese melts. Let set covered for 10 minutes before serving.

Serves; 4

CRUSTLESS QUICHE LORRAINE

10 *breakfast strips, cooked and crumbled

¼ c onion, finely chopped   ¼ c oil

1 c shredded cheese   4 eggs

1 can milk   salt and pepper

¼ t sugar   1/8 t cayenne pepper

Sprinkle strips, cheese and onions in a 9 inch pie plate. Mix remaining ingredients until well blended and pour over the strips. Microwave on high for 9 minutes. Let stand for 10 minutes before serving.

Serves; 6

VEGETABLES/SIDES
SWEET POTATO GRATIN

7 T butter	1 c orange juice
½ c brown sugar	1t. ginger
Nutmeg, pinch	salt & pepper
1 12oz can crushed pineapple	
4 oz sweet potatoes, peeled & sliced	

Combine all ingredients and place in casserole dish. Bake at 350 degrees for 45 minutes.

VEGETABLE PLATTER

English peas	cucumber slices
String beans, sliced	avocado, sliced
Carrots, sliced	asparagus
Green olives	black olives
Romaine lettuce	oil & vinegar dressing

Note: amounts depend on the number to be fed.

Arrange veggies on a large serving platter. Serve with salad dressing and favorite crackers.

Martha Bethea

FRIED SQUASH

6 medium yellow squash	onion, chopped
2 eggs, beaten	salt & pepper
½ t *McCormick seasoning	¼ c oil
1 c. Italian bread crumbs	

Cook squash in water until tender, drain and mash add bread crumbs and seasonings. Form into small patties. Roll patties into beaten eggs then cover with bread crumbs. Fry in vegetable oil until brown on both sides.

Serves: 6-8   Mary Alford

FRIED GREEN TOMATOES

6 medium green tomatoes
½ c bread crumbs
½ t. *McCormick seasoning

2 eggs
½ t. salt
oil

Slice tomatoes. Beat eggs with seasoning. Season the sliced tomatoes then dip in egg mixture then into crumbs, back again in eggs then into crumbs then fry in a skillet with hot oil on both sides until delicately brown.

Florine Tyler

GARLIC ROAST MASH POTATOES

6 cloves garlic, roasted
5-6 lg. white potatoes, cooked
Salt & pepper

1 pt. sour cream

4 T. olive oil

Roast garlic in olive oil in oven for 20 minutes or in microwave for 5 minutes. Mash potatoes, and then add the roasted garlic and seasoning. Sprinkle with parsley and paprika.
Serves: 8

Florine Tyler

VEGETABLES
STUFFED PATTY-PAN SQUASH

4 slices *breakfast strips, cooked
4 patty-pan squash
½ c onion, chopped
½ c milk

¾ c breadcrumbs
½ c butter

Cook squash in boiling water for 15 minutes. Drain and cool. From the stem end cut a small slice, scoop out the center leaving a ½ "rim. Sauté' onion in butter then adds crumbs, milk and reserved squash. Fill the squash cups and place in a casserole dish. Place breakfast strips on top and bake at 350 degree for 25 minutes.
Serves: 4

HARVARD CARROTS

2 lbs carrots

1 ½ T cornstarch

¼ c water

½ c sugar

¼ c vinegar

¼ c butter

Cut carrots into ½ inch slices and cook covered in large saucepan with small amount of water for 15 minutes. Combine sugar and cornstarch in a small saucepan, add vinegar and water. Cook over medium heat until thickened. Add carrots, sauce and butter and cook over heat until thoroughly heated.

Betty G. Perry

TANGY VEGETABLES

1 c. mayo

3 T. lemon juice

1 t. Worcestershire sauce

1 t. garlic salt

Hot pepper, dash

1 pkg. frozen French green beans

1 pkg. frozen lima beans

1 pkg. frozen English peas

2 hard boiled eggs

2 t lemon juice

¼ t garlic salt

1 t. mustard

Combine all sauce ingredients, heating and stir over low heat until just hot. Cook vegetables according to package directions, drain and mix. Pour hot sauce over vegetables and serve.

Serves; 8

Naomi Thompson

SQUASH DELIGHT

3 med. zucchini, sliced

2 cloves garlic, minced

2 med onions, chopped

1 28oz can crushed tomatoes

1 T olive oil

salt & pepper

1 T *McKay's

In medium saucepan place olive oil and onions. Heat until onions are translucent. Reduce heat and add garlic and cook for 2 minutes more. Add zucchini and stir well and frequently. Add tomatoes and seasoning, reduce heat and simmer for 15 minutes. Add salt and pepper to taste.

Serve hot over a bed of brown rice.

Serves: 6   Edna Farmer

VEGETABLES
SQUASH CASSEROLE

1 lb zucchini squash

1 c. cheese, shredded

1 c. crushed crackers

3 eggs

¾ t. oregano

1lb summer squash

1 onion, chopped

2 T butter

¾ t. salt

Coarsely grate unpeeled squash. Sauté' onion in butter. Combine all ingredients. Bake in a buttered 9x12x2 inch loaf pan. Bake in a 375 degree oven for 45 minutes, cut into squares to serve.

Serves: 8-10   Edna Farmer

ZUCCHINI IN SOUR CREAM

6 sm. Zucchini squash

1 T. butter

½ t. salt

2 T. cheese, grated

2/3 c. sour cream

¼ c. cheese, grated

3T. wheat bread crumbs

Cut squash into slices, simmer in small amount of water until fork tender. Drain and place in a 8" pie pan. In a saucepan combine sour cream, butter, ¼ c cheese and salt, heating until well blended. Pour over zucchini. Top with bread crumbs and cheese. Bake at 375 degrees for 10 minutes or until crumbs are golden. Let stand 5 minutes before serving.

Serves: 4-6   Betty G. Perry

ZUCCHINI CHIP CASSEROLE

3 T. butter

1 clove garlic, crushed

2 lbs zucchini, grated

½ c milk

½ c potato chips, crushed

1 onion, sliced

1 ½ t. salt

2 eggs

1/3 c. cheese, grated

paprika

Saute' onion slices and garlic in butter until tender, adding grated zucchini and salt. Cover and cook for 5-10 minutes, then combine the cheese, egg and milk and pour into casserole and sprinkle with crushed potato chips and paprika. Bake in a 350 degree oven for 25-35 minutes.

Serves: 6   Annie flowers

CREAMED SPINACH

2 pkg. frozen spinach   ½ c. sour cream

1 can mushroom soup

1 can *French's fried onions, crumbled or crumbs

Combine all ingredients and place in oiled casserole. Top with crumbled onions or crumbs. Bake until heated through, about 20 minutes in a 350 degree oven.

Serves: 10   Betty G. Perry

VEGETABLES
SWEET POTATO CASSEROLE

3-4lbs. sweet potatoes

1 c. brown sugar, packed or (1/2c. brown sugar and 2t. Sweet N Low Brown)

1 ½ T cornstarch   ¼ t. *Lite salt(optional)

1 ½ t. cinnamon   1 c. apricot nectar

2 t. orange peel, grated

2 T. liquid *Butter Buds

½ c *Grape-nuts cereal

2 8oz. cans mandarin oranges, drained

Boil potatoes and set aside. Combine sugar, cornstarch, *lite salt and cinnamon in a saucepan. Add apricot nectar and orange rind bring to a boil. Remove from heat Pour sauce over slice peeled sweet potatoes and mandarin oranges that have been placed in a casserole dish(9x12) sprayed with non fat cooking spray. Sprinkle grape-nuts on top. Bake at 350 degrees for 25 minutes.

Serves: 6-8   Naomi Thompson

TURNIP GREENS

2 cans turnip greens	1 onion, chopped
Oil	onion powder
Pinch of salt	pinch of sugar

Sauté' onion and oil in pot add remaining ingredients and enjoy.

Serves: 6-8   Mary Alford

VEGETABLE CASSEROLE

1 can white shoe peg corn, drained

1 can French cut green beans, drained

½ c celery, chopped	½ pt. sour cream
½ c onion, chopped	salt & pepper

¼ c green bell pepper, chopped

1 can cream of celery soup

Mix all ingredients together in large casserole. Sprinkle with topping and bake at 350 degrees for 35 minutes.

Serves: 9-10

Topping:

½ box cheese buttered crackers

½ stick butter, melted

½ c almonds, slivered

Crumble crackers and mix with margarine, add almonds.

Naomi Thompson

FRESH TURNIP GREENS

1 bunch turnip greens with bottoms

Oil	salt
1 onion, chopped	½ c water or broth

Sauté' onion in pot with oil. Add cleaned and rinsed turnip greens and cubed bottoms and salt. Cook for 25 minutes or until the desired tenderness.

Serves: 6-8   Mary Alford

VEGETABLE SIDES
*CHIK N DRESSING

1 pan corn bread, baked

½ c. butter	1 ½-2c broth
1 can mushrooms	1 T broth seasoning

½ c each chopped celery, onion, bell pepper

1 can soy chicken, cut up

Combine all ingredients and bake at 350 for 30 minutes

Serves 6-8   Mary Alford

ROLY-POLY CARROT MARBLES

3 oz cream cheese, softened   1 t. honey

¾ c finely chopped peanuts

1 c cheese, shredded

1 c finely shredded carrots

Combine the first 3 ingredients and blend. Stir in carrots. Chill for 1 hour. Shaped into balls using 1 ½ of mixture for marbles. After rolling each marble in the chopped peanuts, chill until firm.

BAKED CREAMED SPINACH

1 c. cream   ¾ c parmesan cheese

3 c. spinach   ½ t. salt

Nutmeg

Whip cream until stiff. Fold in ½ of cheese, then fold into spinach and blend well. Season to taste. Put into buttered pie plate. Sprinkle ¼ c grated cheese on top. Bake in 375 degree oven until slightly browned.

Serves: 6

QUICK STUFFING LOAF

1 onion, chopped   1 c. celery, chopped

3T liquid *Butter Buds (or 3T chicken broth)

3 t. poultry seasoning   3t. sage

1 t oregano   2 slices wheat bread, cubed

1 8 oz can whole kernel corn, drained

1 c. cornmeal

1c. flour   2t. *Sweet N Low or sugar

¼ t. salt   1 c skim milk

¼ t baking powder   3 *Egg Beaters(3/4 c)

Heat oven to 350 degrees. Spray a loaf pan. Cook onion and celery in chicken broth. Stir in spices and mix well Remove from heat. Add bread crumbs and corn and combine all dry ingredients. Add vegetables. Spread evenly into prepared pan. Bake 45 minutes or until tooth pick inserted in center comes out clean. Cool in pan for 15 minutes. Remove from pan and cut into ¾ inch slices. Serve warm.

Serve: 8   Naomi Thompson

SPINACH LOAF

2 c spinach, cooked	1 c. crumbs
1 onion, diced	1 t. salt
½ c nuts, chopped	1/8 t. paprika
2 eggs, beaten	1 T. butter, melted
Milk or stock	

Combine all ingredients adding milk or stock to form a loaf. Place in oiled loaf pan and bake 30 minutes in 375 degree oven.

VEGETABLE SIDES
GREEN BEAN CASSEROLE

3 cans green beans   1 can mushroom

2 cans cream of mushroom soup

1 can *French fried onions

Place drained beans in 9x13 baking dish. Stir mushrooms and liquid into mushroom soup and pour over green beans. Bake in an oven at 350 degrees for 25 minutes. Add onions over top and heat 5-10 minutes longer

Servings: 12   Annie Flowers

YELLOW SQUASH CASSEROLE

2 lbs yellow squash	1 onion, sliced
1 can cream soup	1 c sour cream
Seasonings	1 stick butter
1 pkg. *Pepperidge Farms Dressing Mix	

Boil squash until tender, drain. Sauté onion in butter, add all ingredients and pour into a casserole dish at 350 degrees for 1 hour.

Betty G. Perry

GINGER CARROTS

3 carrots cut into 3x1 strips
1 t. butter   1 t. brown sugar
1/8 t ground ginger

Cook carrots in small amount of boiling water until tender and drain. Melt butter in saucepan stir in ginger and sugar. Cook over low heat stirring constantly then add carrots stirring gently until carrots are coated and hot.

Janet Taylor

TURNIP CASSEROLE

1 ½ lbs. turnips, peeled and sliced
2 T butter   1 onion, sliced
2/3 c celery, chopped   2 t flour
1 c. milk   ½ cheese, grated
Seasonings   3 T breadcrumbs
1 green pepper, diced

Cook turnips in boiling water until tender and drain. Sauté' onion, pepper and celery in butter, then sprinkle with flour and cook for 1 minute longer then add milk, cheese and seasonings. Combine with the turnips and place in a casserole dish covering the top with the bread crumbs, and brown under broiler.
Serves: 4   Betty G. Perry

BROCCOLI CASSEROLE

¼ c. onion, chopped   6T butter
½ c water   2 T flour
8 oz. cheese   ½ c. bread crumbs
2 pkg. broccolis, frozen, chopped
½ c. bread crumbs

Sauté' onion in butter, add flour and cook for 1 minute. Add water, broccoli and cheese stirring well, and add the beaten eggs. Turn into a casserole and place the crumbs over the top and bake at 350 degrees for 30 minutes.
Serves: 8   Joann Barnes

VEGETABLE SIDES
GREEN BEANS & TOMATOES

1 lb fresh green beans

1 bunch green onions, chopped

2-3 T vinegar

2-3 tomatoes, chopped

1/3 c. sour cream

seasonings to taste

Cook green beans, drain and keep warm. Sprinkle chopped onions on top. In bowl mix together sour cream, vinegar and seasonings. Stir in tomatoes and sour cream mixture into beans and serve while warm.

Yields: 4-6 servings

Ethel Bell

PINEAPPLE CASSEROLE

2 cans pineapple chunks

¾ c sugar

1 ½ c. cheese, grated

1 stick butter

5 T plain flour

¾ c. sugar

1 roll *Ritz crackers

Spread pineapple in baking dish, sprinkle on top the flour. Crush the crackers and sprinkle then sprinkle the cheese. Melt the butter and pour over the top. Bake at 350 degrees for 30 minutes.

Florine Tyler

APPLE ZUCCHINI SLAW

½ c vanilla yogurt

2 small zucchini, shredded

1 ½ c apples, chopped ¼ c raisins

1. Ts orange zest

2T sunflower seeds

Combine all ingredients and stir gently to coat.

Servings: 6

Ethel Bell

TOMATOES AND ZUCCHINI

¼ c. butter

1 ½ c. zucchini, sliced

2 cloves garlic, minced

2 cans tomatoes

¾ c crumbs

seasonings

Melt butter in skillet. Add zucchini and garlic. Cook till zucchini is almost tender. Add tomatoes, crumbs and salt. Mix and pour into greased casserole. Bake at 375 degrees for 40 minutes.

Serves: 8

Patricia Davis

HOLIDAY SQUASH

1 butternut squash

1/3 c brown sugar

2 T. coconut extract

seasonings

1c. coconut

2 T butter

Cook squash. Blend. Add other ingredients and bake in casserole dish for 35 minutes at 350 degrees.

Serves: 8

Janet Taylor

GREENS RED POTATOES AND TURNIPS

1 bunch turnip greens   4t. butter

5 red potatoes, cooked and sliced

8 oz. fresh mushrooms, sliced thin

Seasonings to taste

In a medium pot boil turnips greens and potatoes until just tender about 30 minutes. Drain and save the broth. In a saucepan melt butter and saute' mushrooms about 3 minutes. Add potatoes and greens and broth and cook for 15 minutes, season to taste.

VEGETABLE/ SIDES

POTATO N BROCCOLI SUPREME

3 hot mashed potatoes   ¼ c milk

1 3oz pkg. cream cheese   1 egg

2 T butter   1 c. cheese, shredded

1 can *French fried onions

2 pkg. broccoli, thawed and cooked

Whip together first 5 ingredients and season, Place in casserole dish and layer the broccoli and potatoes. Then sprinkle the cheese and remainder of onions on top. Bake uncovered for 10-15 minutes.

CABBAGE AND POTATOES

3 potatoes, cooked, cube unpeeled

4 c. cabbage, chopped, parboiled and drained ¼ t. oil

1 small onion, chopped   5 *Breakfast strips

In skillet add onion and saute' add potatoes, cabbage, sprinkle breakfast strips over the surface. Allow potatoes to become golden on the bottom over medium heat about 20 minutes. Invert skillet over large serving plate and serve.

CRUNCHY-TOP POTATOES

6 T butter   4 lg. potatoes, sliced

¾ c *Kellogg's corn flakes, crushed

1 c. cheese, shredded   salt and pepper

Preheat oven to 375 degrees. Place melted butter in casserole. Place sliced potatoes in melted butter coating well. Mix remaining ingredients and sprinkle on top of the potatoes. Bake 30 minutes or until potatoes are done and are crisp.

CAULIFLOWER BROCCOLI WITH HERB SAUCE

2 baby cauliflowers   1 broccoli

Salt and pepper

Cut cauliflower and broccoli into florets and cook in salted water for 8 minutes. Place in a casserole.

HERB SAUCE:

8 T. olive oil   4 T. butter

2 t. ginger root, grated   salt & pepper

5T. cheese, grated

5 T cilantro, chopped

Juice and rind of 2 lemons

Combine all ingredients except cheese in a small saucepan until butter is melted. Pour over broccoli and cauliflower, then sprinkle with the cheese. Place in broiler for 1-3 minutes or until cheese is bubbly or golden.

Serves: 4-6   Monique Perry Nervis

VEGETABLE SIDES

BEANS N LEMON HERB SAUCE

2 lbs. mixed green beans, cooked

2 T lemon juice	salt and pepper
1 ½ c. broth	6 T. light cream
4 T flour	½ c butter
3 T. mixed herbs	

Melt flour and butter and cook for 1 minute, add broth and bring to a boil. Remove from heat, add herbs and lemon juice. Pour over the beans.

Serves : 4   Monique Perry Nervis

LIMA BEAN CASSEROLE

2 c. cheese, grated	2/3 c. evap. Milk
½ T mustard	2 med. tomatoes
2 c. lima beans, cooked	salt & pepper

Combine cheese, milk and mustard. Cook and stir over hot water until cheese melts and sauce is smooth. Place lima beans in a casserole dish and cover with sauce. Top with tomato slices, salt &pepper and remaining sauce. Bake at 375 degrees for 25 minutes or until lightly browned and bubbly on top.

SPINACH MASHED POTATOES

6-8 Lg. potatoes, cooked and mashed

¾ c. sour cream	1 t. sugar
1 stick butter	salt & pepper
2 t chives, chopped	¼ t. dill leaves

1 10oz pkg. spinach, cooked

1 c. cheese, shredded

To the potatoes add sour cream, sugar, butter, salt and pepper and beat with mixer until light and fluffy. Add chives, dill and drained spinach. Place in casserole and sprinkle with cheese. Bake at 400 degrees for 20 minutes, delicious.

HOT GERMAN POTATO SALAD

8 med potatoes	8 *Breakfast strips
1 onion, chopped	¼ c. oil
3 T. flour	¼ c. sugar
Salt and pepper	½ t. celery seed
1 c. water	1/3 c. vinegar

Pierce potatoes with fork and microwave for about 12 minutes, and then slice. Cut strips in pieces and place in casserole with onion and oil, cover and cook for 4-5 minute. Stir in flour, sugar, celery seed, salt and pepper, then microwave for 3 minutes. Stir in salt, pepper and vinegar and microwave for 5 minutes, stirring until smooth. Add potatoes and strips and stir.

Serves; 8-10

VEGETABLE/ SIDES
FLORENTINE NOODLES

½ c. onion, chopped   ½ c sour cream

1pkg. frozen spinach, chopped

1/8t.nutmeg   salt and pepper

1 can cream of celery soup

2 c. noodles, cooked   dash cayenne

½ c. Parmesan cheese

Place onion in a casserole dish and microwave covered for 1 minute. Add spinach and microwave for 5 minutes. Stir in soup, sour cream, cheese, salt and pepper, nutmeg and cayenne. Cover and microwave for 8 minutes. Add hot noodles, toss to coat.

*2c. cubes *wham can be a delightful addition*

MAKE AHEAD MASHED POTATOES

6 medium potatoes   ½ c. sour cream

1 ½ c cottage cheese   salt and pepper

1/8 t. garlic powder   2t. Dried chives

Butter   parmesan cheese

Paprika

Peel and quarter potatoes. In casserole combine potatoes and ½ c. water, cover and microwave on high for 15 minutes or until very tender, drain. Transfer potatoes to a bowl and beat with electric mixer on low speed. Add cottage cheese, sour cream, garlic powder, chives, salt and pepper beating until smooth. Turn into a greased casserole, brush the top with butter and parmesan cheese and a sprinkle of paprika.

QUICK-FIX POTATO SALAD FOR 20

1 24 oz. pkg. frozen hash browns with onions and peppers

1 ½ c. celery, chopped   salt & pepper

1 pt. sour cream with chives

2/3 c. mayo   1T. mustard

3 hard cooked eggs, chopped

In covered 4 qt. saucepan, cook potatoes with onions and peppers in large amount boiling water 6-8 minutes. Drain into large bowl, combine cooked potatoes with celery and set aside.

DRESSING:

In small bowl stir together sour cream dip, mayo, sugar, vinegar and salt and pepper, toss gently; fold in chopped eggs and add to potato mixture. Cover and chill.

OVEN- FRIED POTATOES

4 lg. baking potatoes, unpeeled

¼ c. oil   2T. Parmesan cheese

Dash garlic powder   salt and pepper

Cut potatoes lengthwise into wedges. Place skin side down in 13x9x2 inch pan. Combine remaining ingredients and brush over potatoes, bake at 375 degrees for 1 hour. Turn potatoes twice during baking process.

VEGETABLE /SIDES
SWEET –TATER CASSEROLE

Medium sweet potatoes, canned or fresh

1 can Bartlett pear halves   ½ c. .butter

1 c. maple syrup

Dash cinnamon & nutmeg

If potatoes are canned, drain, if fresh cook in boiling water until tender. Peel, slice as desired. Combine butter, syrup, cinnamon and nutmeg. Arrange potatoes and drain pears in a shallow buttered casserole. Pour syrup mixture over all and bake at 350 degrees for 35-45 minutes or until glazed, basting a few times in casserole.

POTATO SOUP

4c water or broth   3 potatoes

1 onion, chopped   3T. butter

½ c celery, chopped   1c. milk

In large Dutch oven place sliced potatoes and water, boil until tender; add other ingredients and cook for 20 minutes.

CREAMY CHIVE-STUFFED POTATOES

8 lg. potatoes, boiled with skins

5 hard boiled eggs, chopped

3 sticks celery, diced   ½ c pickle relish

1 onion, minced   1 bell pepper, chopped

¼ c. mustard   2 T. mayo

Cube potatoes and combine all ingredients. Chill

HASH BROWN POTATOES

5 c. potatoes, cooked and cubes

1/3 c. butter   salt & pepper

1 t. onion, minced

Heat butter in skillet and brown potatoes, stirring constantly. Add remaining ingredients and cook well. Sprinkle parsley on top.

PARTY POTATO SALAD

1 2lb. bag frozen hash brown potatoes

1 can cream of potato soup

salt & pepper   paprika

1 can cream of celery soup

½ c. sour cream   1 c. cheese, shredded

½ c. onion green pepper, chopped

½ c. onion, chopped

Combine soups with softened cream cheese. Add sour cream, pepper, onion and seasonings. Put potatoes in 3 qt. baking dish, pour soup mixture over potatoes and stir. Spread out evenly. Sprinkle with cheese. Bake at 325 degrees for 1 ½ hours.

OVEN FRIED SWEET POTATOES

6 med. sweet potatoes   ½ c. oil

Sugar(optional)

Preheat oven to 450 degrees. Cut potatoes in ½ inch pieces. In a bowl coat all sides with oil and arrange on a baking sheet not touching. Bake at 350 degrees for 30 minutes, turning once. Sprinkle with sugar if desired.

VEGETABLE/SIDES
QUICK POTATOES

5 lg. potatoes, sliced   ¼ c. butter

¾ c. cheese, shredded

3 T parmesan cheese

Place potatoes in casserole, pour butter over potatoes and sprinkle with the cheeses. Bake covered at 475 degrees for 25 minutes.

SQUASH MEDLEY

1 onion, chopped   2 tomatoes, quartered

½ lb cheese, grated   salt & pepper

1 green pepper, chopped

½ lb. fresh mushrooms, sliced

4 med zucchini, sliced thin

4 medium yellow squash, sliced thin

1 pkg. frozen Chinese pea pods

In a large skillet, sauté' onion and green pepper until onions and green are tender. Add mushrooms and sauté' a minute longer. Add zucchini, yellow squash, ¼ c. water and salt to taste. Cover and steam approximately 10 minutes, checking a few times and stirring to combine. When vegetables are tender, add pea pods. Stir and cover again for 1-2 minutes. Sprinkle grated cheese on top of vegetables and garnish with tomato quarters. Serve from skillet.

Serves: 8   Janet Taylor

TOMATO PUDDING

10 oz can tomato puree	½ c hot water
½ c brown sugar	½ c. brown sugar
½ t. salt	2c. bread crumbs
1/3 c butter	

Add all ingredients except bread crumbs. Place bread crumbs in oiled casserole and cover with tomato mixture. Bake uncovered at 350 degrees for 30 minutes.

Serves: 4-6   Martha Bethea

CORN PUDDING

1 can creamed style corn	1 stick butter
1 pkg. corn bread mix	2 eggs
1 8oz. container sour cream	

Mix together and pour into casserole dish, bake at 350 degrees for 45 minutes.

CREAMY RICE PUDDING

1-2 c. milk	¾ c sugar
½ c rice, cooked	dash of salt
1 egg	1 t. cornstarch
1 t. vanilla	

Combine all ingredients and into oiled baking dish, bake at 300 degrees for 30 minutes.

VEGETABLES/RICE
GLORIOUS RICE PUDDING

1c. rice, cooked	¼ c raisins
3c. milk	1 egg
¼ c sugar	1/4t. vanilla
Cinnamon sugar	
1 pkg. vanilla pudding (not instant)	

Mix all ingredients and stir constantly until mixture comes to a boil. Spoon into dessert dishes and sprinkle top with cinnamon sugar.

Chill and serve cold.

Serves: 6

HARVARD BEETS

2 cans beets, sliced	2T. sugar
1 T. corn starch	1 cinnamon stick
Dash of allspice	½ c. vinegar
1 l. onion, sliced	

Mix sugar, corn starch, vinegar, allspice and juice from the beets in a saucepan and heat until it starts to thicken, add beets and cinnamon then heat I minute more. Serve warm or cold.

COLLARD GREENS

1 lg. bunch collard greens, chopped

1 lg. onion, chopped

Peppers, chopped

¼ c.oil   1 pkg. onion soup mix

Seasonings to taste

½ c water

Sauté' onions and peppers in oil, mix soup mix in water ad add all ingredients to large stock pot and cook for 30-45 minutes.

DESSERTS

Orange Cookies

1 1/3 c. flour	½ t. baking powder
¼ t. baking soda	1/3 c sugar
6 T. butter	1 egg
1/3 c buttermilk	1 T. orange zest
2 T. orange juice	Orange frosting

Stir together flour, baking powder and soda; set aside. Beat together sugar, butter the add egg, beat until fluffy. Beat in buttermilk, orange zest and orange juice; add dry ingredients and beat until combined. Drop by teaspoonfuls onto ungreased cookie sheets. Bake at 350 degrees for 10-13 minutes. Cool then frost.

ORANGE FROSTING:

Beat together 2 cups confectioner's sugar, 3 teaspoons of orange zest and 3 T. orange juice to make a spreadable thick frosting.

FAVORITE SWEET POTATO PIE

2 ¼ c sweet potato, mashed	
¾ c sugar	½ c brown sugar, packed
½ c. instant vanilla pudding	
¾ c evaporated milk	2 eggs
6 t butter	1t. cinnamon
1 ½ t. vanilla extract	
1 prepared pie crust	

Combine all ingredients in large bowl and blend well. Pour into the 9" unbaked pie crust and bake 40-45 minutes at 350 degrees. Let cool garnish with whipped cream topping.

FAVORITE STICKY PIE CRUST

1 pkg. yellow cake mix   3 T. water

1 T. butter

To make a favorite pie crust, combine yellow cake mix, 3 T water and 1 T butter and spread over a 9" pie pan.

CINNAMON BUNS

1 box bread mix   1c. buttermilk

1 egg   ¼ stick butter, melted

1 pkg. caramel   1 c. pecans

½ c. raisins   ½ c sugar

Oil   1pkg. yeast

¼ c. cinnamon

Place the flour and yeast in mixing bowl add yeast. In microwave heat buttermilk to very warm, then add to the flour mixture and continue to knead the dough. Then add butter and eggs and beat for 2 minutes more. Then set aside for 30-40 minutes to rise. Prepare the baking pan by oiling hen spread a layer of pecans and a layer of melted caramel.

Punch dough down and roll out on floured surface then sprinkle with sugar, cinnamon and raisins. Start rolling up one end in jelly roll style until completely rolled. Take a sharp knife and slice the dough about every 1 ½ inch. Take each slice and place in the pan and allow to rise for 40 minutes. Then bake at 400 degrees for 15-20 minutes. When browned remove from heat and wait 10 minutes and place a platter over and invert. Now remove the pan and enjoy and expect compliments. For variations I use a Christmas tree pan and cherries for decorative effects.

DESSERTS

DESSERTS

Zucchini Cookies

1 c. zucchini, grated

1 c sugar

½ c. butter

1 egg

2 c. flour

1 t. cinnamon

½ t. nutmeg

¾ t. baking powder

½ t. baking soda

¾ c. pineapple, crushed

1 c. nuts, chopped

1 c. raisins

Cream sugar, butter and eggs. Add zucchini and pineapple. Stir in dry ingredients; stir in nuts and raisins. On greased cookie sheet drop by spoonfuls. Bake at 375 degrees for 15 minutes or until no imprint is left when the cookie is press down. These cookies do not brown on top. While still warm, glaze with a thin coat of frosting or glaze.

Anne Flowers

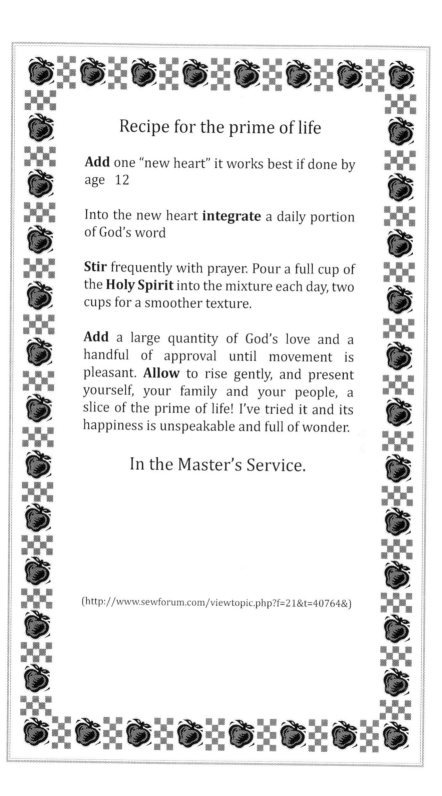

Recipe for the prime of life

Add one "new heart" it works best if done by age   12

Into the new heart **integrate** a daily portion of God's word

Stir frequently with prayer. Pour a full cup of the **Holy Spirit** into the mixture each day, two cups for a smoother texture.

Add a large quantity of God's love and a handful of approval until movement is pleasant. **Allow** to rise gently, and present yourself, your family and your people, a slice of the prime of life! I've tried it and its happiness is unspeakable and full of wonder.

In the Master's Service.

(http://www.sewforum.com/viewtopic.php?f=21&t=40764&)

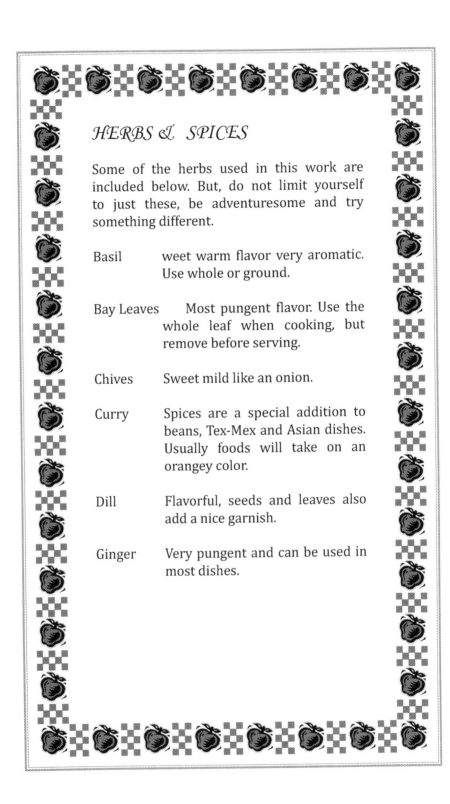

HERBS & SPICES

Some of the herbs used in this work are included below. But, do not limit yourself to just these, be adventuresome and try something different.

Basil   weet warm flavor very aromatic. Use whole or ground.

Bay Leaves   Most pungent flavor. Use the whole leaf when cooking, but remove before serving.

Chives   Sweet mild like an onion.

Curry   Spices are a special addition to beans, Tex-Mex and Asian dishes. Usually foods will take on an orangey color.

Dill   Flavorful, seeds and leaves also add a nice garnish.

Ginger   Very pungent and can be used in most dishes.

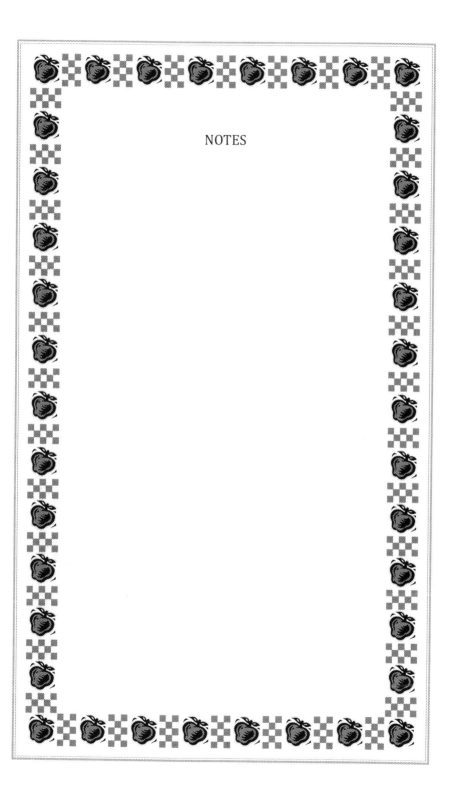

NOTES

Mint	Aromatic and cool. Serve with beverages and many desserts.
Oregano	Strong flavor, adds a taste of Italy to dishes.
Paprika	Red pepper spice, used as a garnish to many dishes.
Parsley	Beautiful when used fresh, use it to garnish and in most other dishes
Sage	Gives meat dishes and stuffing's the sausage taste.
Thyme	Adds that extra touch to your dish.

Spices add the extra touch of love to all dishes.

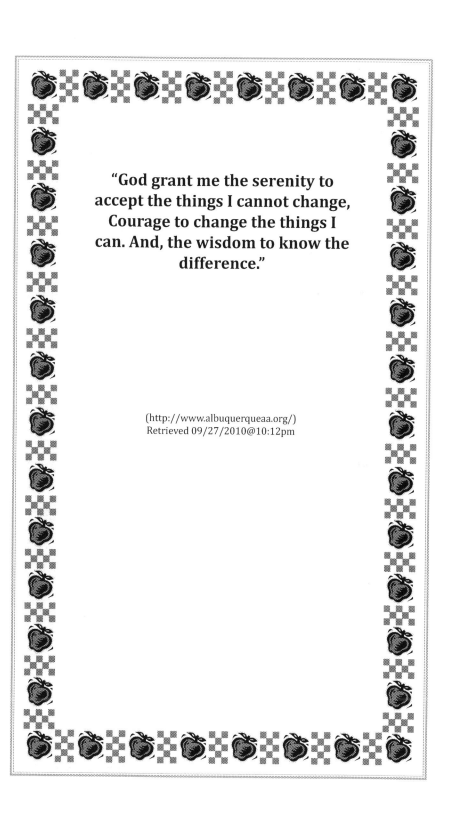

"God grant me the serenity to accept the things I cannot change, Courage to change the things I can. And, the wisdom to know the difference."

(http://www.albuquerqueaa.org/)
Retrieved 09/27/2010@10:12pm

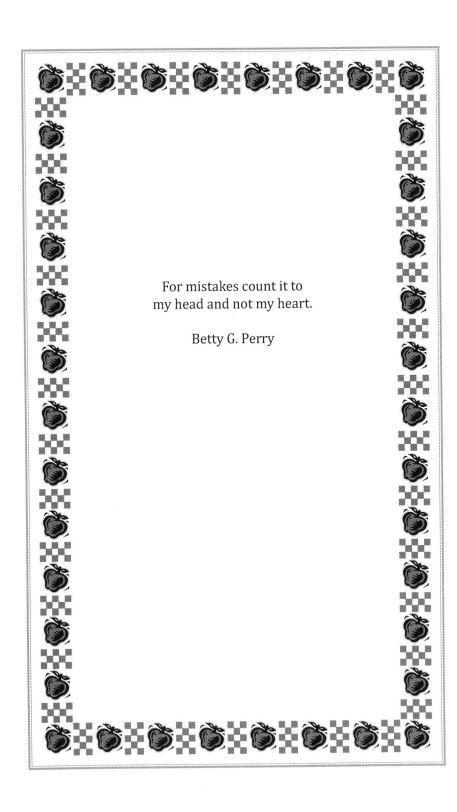

For mistakes count it to
my head and not my heart.

Betty G. Perry

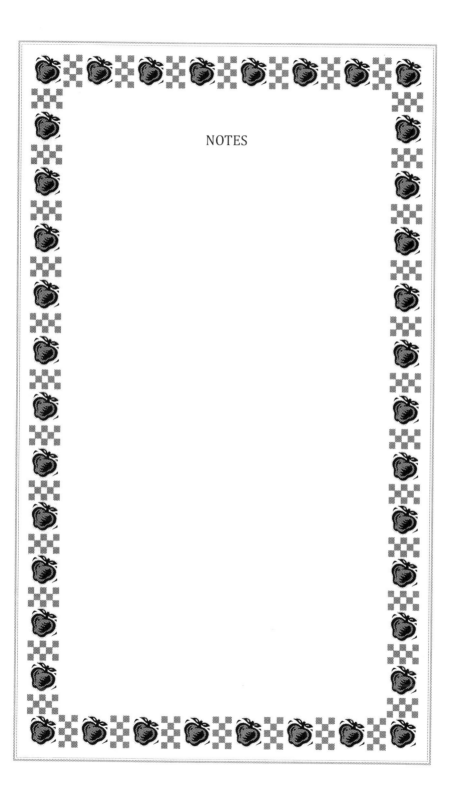

NOTES

NOTES

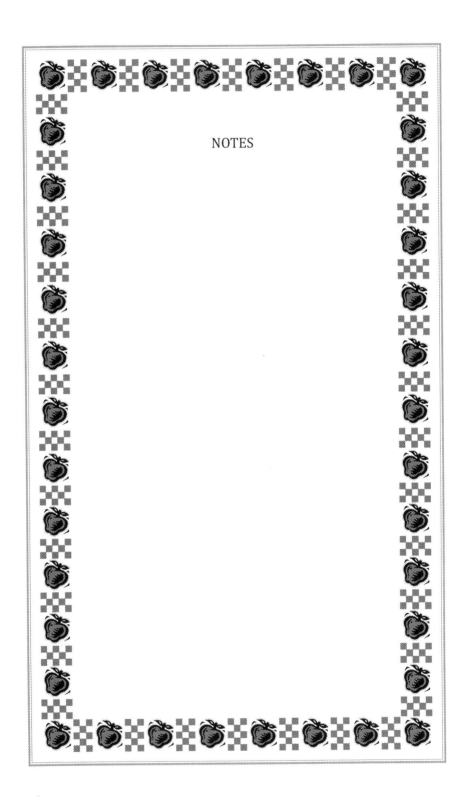